Offering
from the
Conscious Body

ALSO BY JANET ADLER

Arching Backward:
The Mystical Initiation of a Contemporary Woman

Offering
from the
Conscious Body

The Discipline of Authentic Movement

JANET ADLER

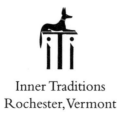

Inner Traditions
Rochester, Vermont

Inner Traditions
One Park Street
Rochester, Vermont 05767
www.InnerTraditions.com

Copyright © 2002 by Janet Adler
Woodcuts by Philip Buller

Library of Congress Cataloging-in-Publication Data
Adler, Janet.
Offering from the conscious body : the discipline of
Authentic Movement / Janet Adler.
p. cm.
Includes bibliographical references.
ISBN 0-89281-966-9
1. Movement, Psychology of—Religious aspects. 2. Dance—Religious aspects.
3. Spiritual life. I. Title.
BL625.94 .A35 2002
616.89'1655—dc21
2002068520

Printed and bound in the United States at Lake Book Manufacturing, Inc.

10 9 8 7 6 5 4 3 2 1

This book was typeset in Bembo with Apolline as the display font

To my mother
Posy Woolf Adler

my first witness
my first blessing

Contents

Acknowledgments

I extend gratitude to every mover and witness who has worked in my presence. Each of you is my teacher. Your work is the bone of this book. People's experiences in the book evolve from a combination of gestures and words which I have had the privilege of seeing and hearing, and of my own experience and imagination.

I am grateful for the teachings within mystical texts in Jewish, Buddhist, and Hindu traditions. I am grateful for the work of William Condon and his development of the natural history approach within the study of non-verbal communication, for the work of Marion Chace and her trust in the life of spirit manifest in the body, for D. W. Winnicott's concept "the good enough mother," for Carl Jung's development of the concepts of personal and collective unconscious and conscious realms.

Julia Gombos, I am deeply grateful for your presence, for the uniqueness of your commitment to the specific development of this discipline throughout the past thirteen years, beginning as my student, then becoming my assistant, and now as my colleague and friend. Thank you for your infinitely patient and tenacious word by word attention to the creation of this book.

The writing of the book and the development of the discipline have become inseparable. For greatly valued support at specific times, thank you Elias Amidon, Linda Aaron-Cort, Joan Chodorow, Harriet Finkelstein, Lynn Fuller, Lizbeth Hamlin-Haims, Neala Haze, Barbara Holifield, David Mars, Andrea Olsen, Patrizia Pallaro, Karen Pando-Mars, Marsha Perlmutter-Kalina, Nora Riley, Karen Rosen, Fu Schroeder, Allegra Snyder, Sox Sperry, Tina Stromsted, Russell Sutter, Karen Truehart, and Lisa Tsetse.

For the offerings of text, in full and edited form, I am grateful to Jeanne Castle, Rusa Chiu, Carol Fields, Cheri Forrester, Annie Geissinger, Jesse Geller, Wendy Goulston, Susan Knutson, Gaye Lagana, Emma Linderman, Julie Miller, Kathee Miller, Shira Musicant, Roz Parenti, Noelle Poncelet, Maggie Tuteur, and Joan Webb.

For your recent committed participation in the discipline, and to some, for your contribution of specific gestures or words, thank you Ellen Emmet, Forest Franken, Loren Olds and Soraia Jorge, Eleni Levidi, Caroline Heckman Liebman, Bill McCully. Thank you Keren Abrams, Silvia Antonini, Marianne Bachmann, Janice Beard Bull, Amrita Carmichael Davidson, Dana Davis, Joan Davis, Susan DeGroat, Annie Deichmann, Tirza Dembo, Teresa Escobar, Christine Evans, Leslie French, Winnie Ganshaw, Marie Elena Garcia, Celine Gimbrere, Harriet Glass, Frauque Glaubitz, Eilla Goldhahn, Rosa Maria Govoni, Irmgard Halstrup, Linda Hartley, Almut Hepper Kirchhofer, Susanne Hofler, Erika Kletti-Ranacher, Benna Kolinsky, Judith Koltai, Leslie Kotin, Fran Lavendel, Julie Leavitt Kutzen, Jackie Mayer-Ostrow, Susan McKenna, Moriah Moser, Barbara Najork, Kedzie Penfield, Marcia Plevin, Heli-Maija Rajaniemi, Paula Sager, Ida Rosa Schaller, Cornelia Schmitz, Julia Shiang, Noga Shomut, Yehudit Silverman, Anke Teigeler, Betina Waissman, and Anna Weatherhogg.

Thank you Susan Davidson, my editor, for generous and sustained attention to the development of this manuscript, to Rachel Goldenberg, and to every other person at Inner Traditions who has so thoroughly and graciously helped to publish this offering.

Thank you Elaine Buller and Thea Goldstine for your wise, skilled, and loving editing of the manuscript.

To my sons, I am deeply grateful for your sensitivity and skills in building the studio where I have the privilege of working, where this book unfolds. Thank you, Joshua, for your light and truth in holding each word with me. Thank you, Paul, for your clarity and depth in envisioning the concept of the cover design with me.

To my husband, Philip, I am deeply grateful for your loving presence as my continuous witness as the discipline unfolded day by day, year by year, as this book developed word by word. Thank you for the beauty of the woodcuts inside and the painting on the cover, for all visible and invisible ways in which you have helped me to bring this book into fruition. Thank you for the gift, your offering of your carved, marble bowl.

In Gratitude to Mary Whitehouse, 1911–1979

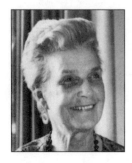 Mary Whitehouse, a student of Martha Graham and Mary Wigman, first became a professional dancer and then a teacher of dance with a developing interest in the inner life, and subsequently in Jungian thought. It was Mary, in her strong and spirited presence, who brought the public relationship between the dancer and the audience into the privacy of the studio. Her early modern dance students learned how to distinguish between performing and moving from an impulse, discovering authentic movement in her presence. Mary's knowledge of body consciousness lies at the core of what has become the phenomenon of mover consciousness.

Words of Mary Whitehouse

"My primary interest might have to do with process not results, that it might not be art I was after but another kind of human development. . . .Whatever it was, we were traveling away from dance. I had to call it movement. . . . For the dance to open out, for it to become more than ourselves in our little, difficult lives, we have to let ourselves be touched, moved."

"When the movement was simple and inevitable, not to be changed no matter how limited or partial, it became what I called 'authentic'—it could be recognized as genuine, belonging to that person."

"There is necessary an attitude of inner openness, a kind of capacity for listening to one's self. . . . It is made possible only by concentration and patience. . . .The kinesthetic sense can be awakened and developed . . . but I believe it becomes conscious only when the inner, that is, the subjective connection is found."

"'I am moved' . . . is a moment when the ego gives up control . . . allowing the Self to take over moving the physical body as it will. It is a moment of unpremeditated surrender that cannot be explained, repeated exactly. . . .The core of the movement experience is the sensation of moving and being moved. . . . "

This material can be found in Patrizia Pallaro, ed. *Authentic Movement: Essays by Mary Starks Whitehouse, Janet Adler and Joan Chodorow* (London: Jessica Kingly, 1999).

In Gratitude to John Weir, 1913

Dr. John Weir's work as a psychologist and as a master teacher of human development emerges from the lineage of Sigmund Freud, Wilhelm Reich, and Carl Rogers. John's deep understanding of somatic phenomenology, interpersonal relationships, and psychodynamic theory grounds his fluid and innovative work with groups. The core of his gift to me is the foundation of what has become the phenomenon of witness consciousness.

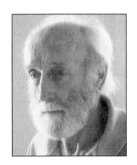

Words of John Weir

"The emphasis is more on the process of Becoming than on the content of Being."

"Our existential aloneness is the precondition for everything we feel, do and think.

"Self-discipline is a necessary aspect of spontaneity and freedom of expression."

"The only way out is in and through." [Personal communication]

"Personal growth is a continuing process of self-differentiation. . . . This process is an orderly one."

"I am the sole authority over my inner life and feelings."

"All my experience takes place solely within me, within the confines of my body. It occurs continuously, from moment to moment. I live only in the here and now."

"The aim of sensory exploration, physical contact, and expressive movement is to reacquaint the participant with his body and its processes. The conscious management of these processes demands a high degree of control and a type of self-discipline that approaches a form of asceticism."

"It is essential that participants share their experiences with others. . . . The sharing . . . performs a kind of witnessing. . . . Witnessing seems to be extremely important in connection with many ritualistic and ceremonial activities. Witnessing, and sharing for that matter, seem[s] to validate the event and to give it and the participant public sanction and acceptance."

This material can be found in Bennem, Bradford, Gibb and Lippitt, ed. *The Laboratory Method of Changing and Learning* (Palo Alto: Science and Behavior Books, 1975).

Preface

When you brush a form clean, it becomes truly what it is.

RUMI

In 1969, in my twenty-eighth year, I experienced the depth of Mary Whitehouse's way of knowing body consciousness and the clarity of John Weir's perception of the self in relationship. Though my encounters with my teachers were brief, the jewel I received from each became the source for the discipline of Authentic Movement, developing within the following three decades of my studio work. This discipline has evolved because of each individual who has committed to it and because of my deep, inexplicable need to track its unfolding.

It is my understanding that it was John Martin, a renowned dance critic and essayist, who was the first person to use the words "authentic movement" in speaking of the dances of Mary Wigman in 1933.

> This class of dance is in effect the modern dance in its purest manifestation. The basis of each composition in this medium lies in a vision of something in human experience which touches the sublime. Its externalization in some form which can be apprehended by others comes not by intellectual planning but by "feeling through" with a sensitive body. The first result of such creation is the appearance of certain entirely *authentic movements.*

It is not surprising that though these words come from the world of dance, authentic movement has become a source from which both therapeutic and mystical experiences manifest. Witnessing the emergence of a discipline with authentic movement reverberating at its center, I have been witnessing the body as a vessel in which healing occurs, a vessel in which direct experience of the Divine is known. As the vessel becomes conscious, it becomes more capable of enduring the darkness and receiving the light of our humanity.

This work has become a discipline because practice has unveiled an inherent order, creating a form with a theoretical ground, revealing a field of study. The discipline of Authentic Movement slowly became apparent as immersion in studio work relentlessly pushed toward the edges of that which we could not yet know. Trusting only what we could know, which was our experience in our bodies, was challenging, at times for me unbearable. Stumbling into clearer seeing in blessed moments was ecstatic. It was as though the form itself was insisting on opening. I repeatedly experienced such a call directly in my body. The tension between the longing to see the emerging form clearly and the longing to surrender to the mysteries of embodiment within it contained potential for transformation of the work, and of the individuals committed to it. In moments of grace, the clarity and the mystery became one.

The architecture of the discipline of Authentic Movement is based on the relationship between a mover and a witness, the ground form. For each, work is centered in the development of the inner witness, which is one way of understanding the development of consciousness. In this discipline the inner witness is externalized, embodied by a person who is called the outer witness. Another person, called the mover, embodies the moving self.

This relationship evolves within the study of three interdependent realms of experience: the individual body, the collective body, and the conscious body. The work is developmental but not linear, as both personal and transpersonal phenomena occur in the practice within each realm. Individuals can enter this evolving practice at any time if experience in another discipline appropriately prepares them.

The first realm concerns the study of the individual body. With a longing to be seen in the presence of a witness, a person moves into the emptiness of the studio with eyes closed, learning to track her movement and her concomitant inner experience. The mover discovers an infinite range of physical movement, sensation, emotion, and thought as embodied experiences happen into consciousness. In this process, there is a discovery of movement that is authentic, truthful. As her inner witness strengthens the mover opens toward a longing to see an other. Becoming a witness, she learns to track another mover's physical movement while becoming conscious of her own sensation, emotion, and thought as she sits in stillness to the side of the space.

Because language bridges experience from body to consciousness, the mover and the witness speak, within their developing relationship, after every round of work, each intending toward the demanding practice of clear articulation. As the work deepens, there is a freedom to directly enter the body and the word, to discover each as sacred.

Practice focused on the collective body, the second realm, concerns still another longing, a longing to participate in a whole, to discover one's relationship to many without losing a conscious awareness of oneself. In this realm of study and practice people bring their experience of the ground form into a circle of movers and witnesses. Here individuals move with eyes closed as members of a moving body and sit in stillness with eyes open as members of a witness circle. In the beginning and ending of each round of work, the circle is empty. As individuals commit to witnessing the emptiness, the vessel strengthens in relationship to the development of embodied collective consciousness.

As the circle expands toward work within the conscious body, the third realm, the form itself becomes more transparent. Personality shifts toward experience of presence, empathy shifts toward compassion, and, in moments of grace, suffering becomes bearable. Practice toward presence develops into moments in which the body as a vessel is experienced as empty.

Another longing, a longing to offer, emerges out of this emptiness. The body moving becomes more transparent, becomes dance, and dance becomes an offering. Words, becoming transparent, transform into poetry, and poetry is an offering. When energetic phenomena, which can be known in the body as direct experience of the Divine, concentrates within and moves through the conscious body, the energy itself becomes an offering—to the mover, to the witness, to our world evolving, to our world longing for consciousness. As the collective receives and, at times, enters the offerings, we are reminded that this discipline grows from ancient ground.

The roots of this work, apparent in all three realms of the discipline, are directly known in dance, healing practices, and mysticism. The dyadic relationship between a mover and a witness most clearly reflects the root system originating in early healing practices, what has come to be understood in the West as a therapeutic container. In many ways, the Western therapist manifests specific and defining qualitites of the ancient rabbis, priests, and shamans who consciously held both the emotional and spiritual lives of individuals, of communities. In the discipline of Authentic Movement, the literal force of moving and witnessing the embodiment of sensation, emotion, and spirit infuses relationship with new ways of knowing the self and the other.

Because of such depth and complexity of the embodied inner life of the mover, the witness, and their developing relationship, at this time it is most appropriate for a teacher of this discipline to be a professionally trained dance/movement therapist or a body-based psychotherapist. Other therapists, meditation teachers, choreographers, political activists, and movement practitioners who include aspects of this discipline in their professional practice can safely strengthen their work by commited practice with a teacher of the discipline. It is essential for a teacher of the discipline of Authentic Movement to have extensive practice and study in personal process within the developmental work of the form. The discipline is always continuing to evolve because of each person who enters it and because of each teacher who offers from her own developing perspective.

The teacher guides the conscious development of relationships between the moving self and the inner witness, between the individual body and the collective body, between the self and the Divine. Being seen and seeing, participating and offering, movers and witnesses return toward themselves as they commit to the rigorous practices of concentration and discernment, as they discover experiences of intuitive knowing, of awe.

This book, my offering, tracks the development of a discipline that I have come to experience as a mystical practice. One way mystical practice can be recognized is when individuals commit toward that which cannot be known by committing to a practice revealing that which can be known—conscious embodiment. In different ancient and contemporary traditions, descriptions of mystical experiences are similar. There is a call toward entering emptiness. With eyes closed and with focus inward, there is an intention toward staying present, toward practicing the art of concentration. There is practice toward the rigor of impeccability in tracking inner experience. There is a longing for a language that could describe direct experience, that which is indescribable. Ritual occurs, becomes necessary. The blessing of clear, silent awareness can become known. There is a longing for daily life to manifest such a blessing, such awareness. Coming into conscious relationship with mystical experiences requires a strong enough inner witness, one which evolves out of an extensive grounding in an embodied awareness practice.

As the discipline of Authentic Movement unfolds, individuals become a part of a woven reality, simultaneously knowing the clarity and aloneness of their separateness and the essential warmth, the compassion emerging from the direct touching with the ones who are near them doing what they are doing. There can be moments in which the graceful blessing of unitive consciousness can be known, a direct experience in which the boundaries describing all relationships, within and without, dissolve.

The
Individual
Body

Developing
Mover
Consciousness

First we must work in our individual body,
without seeking any escape, since this body
is the very place where consciousness connects
with Matter.

THE MOTHER

The Mover

The depth of primordial being is called Boundless.
Because of its concealment from all creatures above
and below, it is also called Nothingness. If one asks,
"What is it?" the answer is, "Nothing," meaning:
No one can understand anything about it. It is negated
of every conception. No one can know anything about
it—except the belief that it exists. Its existence
cannot be grasped by anyone other than it. Therefore
its name is "I am becoming."

KABBALAH

◐ We begin with the study and practice of the mover because we begin life as movers, with no inner witness, with no consciousness. Many of us arrive into adulthood, into practices concerned with the development of consciousness, such as the discipline of Authentic Movement, with some experience of an inner witness, with some consciousness, and with a desire to be present. We arrive with a longing toward a new way of knowing, a new way of experiencing our suffering, our liberation.

In this discipline there are two separate but mysteriously related realms of the mover's work, interpersonal and intrapersonal. It is the awesome and elusive, ever changing relationship between these realms that guides the development of mover consciousness. The interpersonal work concerns the mover's relationship with her outer witness. Because we weren't seen enough or seen with enough acceptance or seen with enough love or seen with enough consciousness, we arrive into adulthood with the longing to be seen by another. There is a felt need, so profound in the West, to be seen as one is, doing what one is doing. Sometimes we arrive because we are ready to deepen our capacity to love, to forgive, to accept ourselves and others. These yearnings are what bring a mover into the presence of a witness.

Though a mover desires to be seen in her own truth by her outer witness, she also, because of her personality, fears being seen. The choice to risk being seen by a witness inevitably includes a willingness to endure the possibility of not feeling seen. In the right circumstance and the right time this risk is essential, because in human development it is only when one does feel seen by another that one can see oneself.

The intrapersonal work concerns the forming of the inner witness. The presence of the outer witness can become a compassionate model for the aspect of the mover that is becoming conscious of her own experience. It is the development of the inner witness that creates the evolution of the mover's consciousness. With growing awareness the mover learns to distinguish between merging with her movement, being in a dialogic relationship to it, and, in moments of grace, knowing a wholeness, feeling no separation between her moving self and her inner witness.

The inner witness learns to accompany the body into the shapes of the moving self, discovering one's truth. The inner witness learns to honor that which the body directly knows. The body is our sensation, our felt emotion. The body is our experience of ourselves, our temple in which the light of our spirit burns. Unconscious worlds, numinous worlds, worlds with high order and worlds with no apparent order can become known within the body, because of the body.

All movements in this discipline must be discovered by the mover. They are not given to her. In the presence of the outer witness, gestures both cultural and idiosyncratic find their way into consciousness, followed by complex and evocative inner experiences, demanding attention from the mover's inner witness. A mover's journey can begin in chaos and evolve into embodied order, clarity, and wisdom. A mover's journey must begin as her own—inevitably, if commitment endures, only to become everywoman's and everyman's.

Now at my desk, here in my studio, I turn and look outside through the window behind me and see the white lilies, first signs of spring. Now turning back, I look inside and across the room, watching light fall into the massive stone vessel in the corner. I remember a moment here last week when I see a mover step onto the wooden floor, leaving the carpet behind, and walk slowly toward the bowl. As she arrives there I see her pant leg slightly brush its rim. She stops and, standing with her feet in light, her right arm gently extends down. In her hand she is holding her white shawl. Silently she drops the shawl to the floor.

In my presence as her witness, the mover, with eyes closed, commits to her longing as she begins a sustained and extensive exploration of the unknown.

Her inner witness:

> I long to be seen
> by you
> and I am afraid
> to be seen
> by you.
> I long to see myself
> more clearly.
> Can I bear
> to see myself
> feel myself, know
> myself?
> Mostly my body

moves
without me
yet I am risking
to actually move
in your presence.
I need you
to see me more clearly
first
so that I can
then see myself.
It is the grace
of clear, silent awareness
for which I long.

"Heneni." Here I am.

It is time to begin. A mover is sitting on her cushion on the carpet, here near the low table. I am the witness, sitting on my cushion across from her, speaking to her now.

Before us is an empty space, shaped by the walls and the floor, by the open, high ceiling, by the door and window frames and the light spilling through them. All of it, all of this emptiness, is a reflection of our potential experience of emptiness within. I invite you to enter this emptiness as a mover. Here the emptiness can fill and empty because of you. Here you can fill and empty because of it.

As you leave your cushion be aware that you will return to it when your experience as a mover is completed. After you move to the edge of the carpet, either before facing the unknown or once you've stepped in, I invite you to make eye contact with me. When our eyes meet we will be consciously connecting in a shared commitment toward the longing to be seen and to see in the presence of each other. We will be marking a gateway in that moment as we formally begin our relationship within the discipline of Authentic Movement.

As the mover in this practice you will step into the emptiness not knowing, not knowing what you will actually do, how you will move. There is no way that either of us can know what you should be doing. Remember, there is no right or wrong way to move. When you are ready, intend toward listening inwardly. Close your eyes to erase the visual world around you, though perhaps you can still sense my presence or where the light is coming in.

It will be here, when you encounter the possibility of making conscious choices, that the practice of discernment begins. You may choose to move or you may wait for an impulse to move. If an impulse arises you may choose to surrender to it, or you may choose to bring your will in relationship to it and say no. What matters more than what you choose is your freedom of conscious choice, creating a developing clarity of your own subjective experience.

Once moving, if you make big movements or you move suddenly or fast you must open your eyes so that you don't hurt yourself. If you find a place in the room that feels correct for you, you can stop there or keep moving. If you stop, you do not have to know why you are stopping or why you are choosing that particular spot. You could be choosing it for rational reasons or because intuitively it welcomes you or calls to you. Or perhaps you are not consciously choosing it, it just happens to be where you are in that moment.

As I am speaking, I see the mover's white shawl draped over her lap, the soft threads of one end just touching the carpet.

Your inner witness might notice many things happening. You might be moving or be still, making a sound or being silent. You might be moving quickly or slowly, with large gestures or small ones. You might notice inner experiences, such as sensations, emotions, or thoughts. Sometimes it is difficult to sort out all of the different kinds of experiences you are having. As a way to begin, I invite you to try to bring your awareness toward what your body is doing. Try to focus primarily on the movement itself. It is here that the practice of concentration begins.

And the practice of discernment continues. At any moment, for any reason, you can choose to open your eyes and either make eye contact with me or not. You can then close them again and keep moving or you can stop and return to your cushion. If you choose, you can keep moving until five minutes have passed. Then I will call your name and ask you to bring your experience to an end.

As I witness you move, I cannot know your experience. I can only know my own experience in your presence. I commit to tracking my experience as best I can. It is my intention, my practice, to notice all that occurs within me as I witness.

When you finish moving and you open your eyes, before you come back to your cushion I invite you to make eye contact with me

again. As we look at each other then, we will be moving back
through the gateway of conscious connection that we marked by
our eye contact as you were entering the space. We will be
acknowledging our commitment to come toward consciousness in
the presence of each other. Then when you are ready, come back to
your cushion.

Now the mover stands and turns toward the emptiness. May I be able:

> *to see what I am ready to see,*
> *to hear what I am ready to hear,*
> *to know what I am ready to know,*
> *and to be as I am.*

Wrapping her shawl around her shoulders, she walks away from me toward
the carpet's edge. Standing there, I see her toes curled around the softness
of the carpet as it meets the hard wooden floor. Now she turns back toward
me and our eyes meet. She closes her eyes and her movement begins. I am
flooded with gratitude for her willingness to trust me enough.

Her inner witness:

> I long
> to move freely
> with no inhibitions.
> but I don't know how.
> I am inhibited
> by this body
> this body
> that I know
> and that I don't know.

I want you
to accept this body
just as it is
but how could you?

I am self-conscious
as I walk
wondering if you
think I am
clumsy
wondering what
you think of me.

Will you like me
if I move
this way or that?
Don't project
all that is unconscious
in your own life
onto mine. Don't
interpret
my being.

I witness the mover for five minutes. It is time for her to bring her experience to an end. I call her name and ask her to open her eyes when she is
ready. We make eye contact and she returns to her cushion.

After moving there are many ways of being. You can choose not to
speak and we can sit together in silence. You can choose to speak of
your arrival here now, what it is you experience coming out of all
of that movement. Or you can choose to open now toward finding
words that are born, moment to moment, from the movement itself.

If you choose this way, try closing your eyes again as you begin discovering words, choosing some of them, surrendering into others, just as you discover, choose, or surrender into the movement itself when you are working in the space. This continuation of your inner focus as you are sitting here on your cushion also makes speaking in the present tense natural. The present tense reminds us, holds us, encourages us to remain in the embodied, moving experience, riding it as it becomes language. Learning to speak experience rather than speaking about it means learning how to speak without abandoning the authenticity of the moving experience.

The shift from moving with eyes closed to talking with eyes open occurs over time. In the beginning, not only speaking in the present tense but speaking with eyes closed helps such a transition to become more seamless. Sometimes a mover, when embarking on the experience of speaking, reenters the gestures in a modified way while sitting here or actually returns to the wooden floor and walks through the movement, talking to me as she goes.

Try now to remember what your body was doing while you were moving, and perhaps the sequence of your movements. After you speak I will tell you as your witness what I saw your body doing, including the sequence of your movements. Together we will articulate a map that names, places, your body moving in time and space. This map is the essential ground from which all of our experiences can become known.

The mover chooses to speak her experience, now closing her eyes.

> Besides milky fragments, I remember only the
> end, when I am lying on my side over there in

front of the bowl. I don't know how long I am
lying there. It feels like a really long time.

I see the mover open her eyes.

I can't remember anything else clearly so I will try
walking it through.

Now she stands and moves out into the space, both closing and opening her
eyes as she tangentially shifts back into some qualities and gestures of her
original movement experience. She is speaking aloud as she moves.

In the beginning, I think I am walking this way,
going first over here toward the stone bowl and
then . . . now I remember . . . as I come down on
all fours like this, I rock? And in the end, I think
I am in front of the bowl, lying down for a long
time.

She returns to her cushion and as I say her name, I offer my experience of
tracking her physical movement.

*I see you stand up, wrapping your shawl around your
shoulders. My gaze follows you as you walk toward the
carpet's edge. Now I see you standing just at that edge
where the carpet meets the floor, your toes curled around
it. You turn back toward me as our eyes meet.*

*Closing your eyes, you step onto the wooden floor and
into the emptiness. I see your toes lightly touch one of
the floor pillows to your right on your way to the bowl.
Yes, I see you walk directly toward the stone bowl.*

*With each step I see your heels lifting up, one by one.
I can see the soles of your feet, the very shape of them.*

*As you arrive at the bowl I see your pant leg slightly
brushing the rim of it. You stop moving and stand. I do
not see any movement. Still, I do not see any movement.
I do not see any movement. Now I see your right hand
pull your shawl from your left shoulder, down and across
your chest, until it slips to the floor.*

The mover remembers.

Yes, I'd forgotten that. I remember now, I pull it
like this off of my shoulder, down across my chest
and drop it on the floor there by the edge of the
bowl.

*Yes, and now directly in front of the bowl, I see you turn
to your left and face back into the room. Your right
shoulder pulls in toward your chest, your body following
downward. I see you land on your hands and knees. I
too remember your rocking. I see you rock forward and
back, forward and back, forward and back . . . three
times. Now your body lands fully on the floor. You are
curled on your right side, with your hand resting on
your cheek. I can see your face. I remember you lying
there and still lying there until I call your name.*

We are both silent for a long time. With her eyes closed and with a new
quality of attention in her voice, in her face, the mover speaks again, gently
moving into the gesture while sitting on her cushion.

I rock on my hands and knees, forward and back,
forward and back, forward and back.

I see tears spilling from the mover's eyes as she speaks. The space between and around us suddenly deepens as we sit together, looking at each other, both receiving her simple and truthful words. Because of the way in which she speaks these words, opening to the fullness of her moving experience, she is filling with emotion. In the absence of a premature struggle to name this emotion, these movement words glisten as the bare bones of what we come to know later as a source of deep suffering. These words, becoming more vibration than symbol, bridge the experience from body to consciousness.

◻ Embodied consciousness requires a study of articulation not only of body but of word. This mover begins speaking with very little consciousness of what she was actually doing. She is mostly merged with her moving self, her inner witness barely aware of her body's movement, at times her inner witness not present at all. Like this woman, many movers remember their movement only as they are reentering the gesture while speaking it into consciousness.

"I rock forward and back, forward and back, forward and back." Here in the first session, after glimpsing a memory of rocking and then hearing me speak the rocking, the mover enters into it briefly on her cushion and then speaks it again. Eventually all of the emerging sensations and emotions embedded within this gesture must be embodied and then named so that they can be integrated into consciousness. But taking time in the beginning of the practice to speak just the physical movement, without such complexities, makes space for the mover to find a way of talking that comes toward the truth of her experience. In doing so she is not reporting about what happened, she is not listing her observations, she instead is finding her way toward speaking that which her body knows.

Naming only the physical movement carves an articulate map, a sculptural one, which grounds all that the mover and witness share. The map reflects a collection of experiences, pools of movements, as they become apparent. In the beginning of the practice, when speaking after moving, a mover is encouraged to create a pool by naming certain physical movements that feel related as well as marking where she is in the room, if she is aware of it. As the practice develops pools are also shaped by experiences of sensations or emotions. Sometimes the movement series is experienced as one long pool because of a particular movement, a quality of movement, a sensation or an emotion that is apparent throughout. Once the pools are remembered and marked, the detail within them often becomes more accessible.

As we name the pools the sequence that unfolds becomes a series of pools. Sometimes there is a transition between two pools that feels important to mark. In this woman's work today, movements concerning her walking to the edge of the carpet, our eye contact, and her subsequent stepping onto the wooden floor might be experienced by her as the first pool. Walking to the stone bowl could be the next pool of gestures. Her movement in front of the bowl, rocking, and then lying down could be another pool. Opening her eyes, looking at me, and returning to her cushion would then be the last pool.

Sometimes a mover cannot begin by tracking and pooling her physical movement because she is filled with sensations or emotions. When this happens my task as the witness/teacher is to help the mover place the fullness of these experiences within the context of a map. Each mover requires a different amount of time to become skilled in tracking different aspects of her work with ease. Movers have different natures, specific ways of experiencing their worlds. One is more emotional, another more kinesthetic, another more thoughtful, imagetic, or tactile. One mover might find tracking emotion quite easy but be more challenged by tracking physical movement. It therefore seems appropriate for the witness/teacher to try to both follow the individual mover's nature, bringing attention to sensation or emotion as it appears most naturally for her, and at the same time to encourage the mover to ground it in physical movement as soon as possible.

The mover learns to keep asking: "Where am I now?" "What am I doing?" And responding: "Here I am. Here I am in front of the bowl, curled on my side, my hand resting on my cheek." Trying to be present for each moment of gesture invites the mover to actually take herself seriously. The mover learns about this new way of experiencing herself as she listens to me, her witness, track her physical movement, taking each of her movements seriously. Doing this I am remembering her, marking, holding each gesture. When I name each gesture in this way the mover can learn that each one of her movements is worthy of being seem. This profoundly simple act of acknowledgment creates a spaciousness early in the development of the practice, before the mover and the witness share more of their experiences.

When moving, clear tracking requires first awareness and then remembering. Being present, aware in the moment, doesn't necessarily mean remembering when the mover opens her eyes and comes back to speak. It is a different process to speak in the present tense now, sitting on the cushion, naming the physical movements from five minutes ago. The intention to remember the precise experience after moving can for some movers result in an awkwardness at first, the effort becoming a distraction from being present while moving. The transition work of speaking the experience with eyes closed, as well as walking through the movements, supports the intention to remember.

Remembering brings language, inviting a consciousness of the experience. Developing this consciousness invites a relationship to what is happening, creating potential for integration. The mover becomes released from the effort to be present in the moments of moving and the effort to remember after moving as integration occurs. When the body is the primary teacher, committed practice develops a capacity to speak what is remembered with eyes open, on the cushion, staying in relationship with the witness.

When the witness tracks the mover's work so carefully, the mover is learning, perhaps feeling, that the witness is in fact present enough. As the mover's trust of the witness presence develops, trust of her own movement can deepen, allowing her to be as she is, to do what she does. She might notice that her witness does not speak her own judgments, her projections, or even her interpretations. The witness is inviting her to bring such complete acceptance toward herself, allowing her inner witness to bring less judgment, projection, or interpretation in relationship to her own experiences.

The mover's choice of words actually helps her to accept, to honor her experience as her own. Sometimes a mover refers to her own body parts using the article *the,* as in "the hands" or "the feet" instead of "my hands," "my feet." As the witness/teacher I suggest saying "my hands, my feet." Every aspect of the body must be claimed, felt, intimately known before, if ever, referred to as hands and feet that have transcended specific identity.

Another way language can keep an experience farther away from the body knowing is when the mover is thinking about what is happening instead of experiencing what is happening. As a result, much of her experience directly known in her body can become obscured. As the witness and the mover accept and include such a natural tendency in the human psyche, the mover learns more about staying within the embodied experience. As this happens, insight, another way of knowing, becomes possible. Insight, which could be called intuitive seeing, exists without intention to understand. The blessing of insight arrives with no effort, one second, minutes, or days following the moving experience. In the meantime the mover experiences an increasingly thoughtful relationship to her work beyond the rigor of the moving/speaking practice.

Often insight occurs in direct relationship to a developing embodied consciousness of a movement pattern. It is not uncommon during the very first movement session for a mover, like this woman, to touch lightly down and into a movement that later, as trust in the relationship with her inner and outer witness strengthens, becomes the vortex of a movement pattern. A movement pattern is a gesture or series of gestures that spontaneously repeats itself. Such a pattern appears as idiosyncratic, with no conscious connection to the knowing self. Born from an unconscious source, as a pattern increasingly manifests, the movement within the pattern becomes more articulate, calling for attention, for a deepening commitment. Repetition of the physical movement becomes apparent first, followed by an awareness of sensation and emotion as time passes.

Because of moving in the presence of a committed outer witness who is honoring, tracking her movement, the mover's inner witness awakens, inviting her into the spiral of developing mover consciousness. As she becomes practiced in noticing and naming the fine details of her movements and the sequence of the pools, she is experiencing a relationship between her moving self and her inner witness. Here her experience of an inner dialogue begins to replace an original merged state.

The mover comes here every week, along the brick path, up the two steps, onto the small deck, and into my studio. She is immersed in strengthening her ability to track her physical movement. She moves and I witness. She moves and I witness. She moves and I witness. Time passes.

I hear the mover's footsteps. I see her pause at the doves' house, looking at the three white birds. As she comes inside, leaving her shoes at the door, she speaks of her pleasure at seeing the bouquet of red poppies on the low table here in front of our cushions. She speaks of her experience of clarity in committing to this practice. As we prepare to begin I remind her that, depending on the length of the first movement time, there could be time for two or three opportunities for moving and dialogue. I continue, offering new guidelines.

As you step once again into the emptiness, continue to bring awareness toward what your body is doing, and now include your awareness of sensation while you are moving. Using the map of your physical gestures as a ground reference, try to bring attention toward receiving your inner experience: what you hear, see with your eyes closed, smell, feel on your skin, or experience kinesthetically as you move. In this particular way of sorting, everything except emotion or thought can be understood to exist within the vastness of the sensory world.

Sensation can precede emotion, informing us about our actual emotional experience, but often we are not aware of such subtle distinctions. For instance, I'm a mover and my heartbeat accelerates, my breath becomes shallow, and my palms are sweaty. Because of my experience of these sensations I know that I am afraid. When you feel a sensation it doesn't matter whether you contain it or whether you express it through movement or sound. It is your intention to choose that matters. It is your developing awareness of your own timing in relationship to opening toward conscious experience of sensation that matters.

As your witness I have been naming your physical movement even when you do not name it first. This is because your body moving is all that I can objectively see. I can see you walk to the bowl. I can see you rock back and forth on your knees. I trust that speaking what I see you doing does not violate your boundaries. But now as we include the task of tracking sensation, if you haven't yet spoken your sensations I do not want to possibly complicate or confuse your inner experience by speaking my own experience of sensation as I witness. Because it is my desire to stay as close as I can to your experience, when you do speak your sensations in relationship to your movement I will offer my experience, but only when it seems resonant with yours.

I see the mover leave her cushion and crawl toward the edge of the carpet, dragging her shawl behind her. The space looms before us wide and high in this particular light. She pauses, looking back at me over her shoulder, and then closes her eyes. Now she stands and walks onto the wooden floor.

Her inner witness:

> I feel
> a new way
> new spaces
> opening inside
> yet oddly familiar
> I'm just me.
> Staying here now
> I must focus
> as I walk.
> Walking I remember
> my child's first steps
> teetering just like me now.
> I'll imagine him in the stone bowl
> see him playing
> safely contained
> and now I can be here.
> Teetering, rocking

> I am coming nearer to myself.
> I remember
> an old way
> in new spaces
> opening inside
> oddly familiar
> I'm just me.

I am the witness speaking now and ten minutes have passed. It is time to bring your experience to an end. Take as much time as you need for transition.

After we make eye contact and the mover returns to her cushion, I suggest that she briefly name the pools and then return to each one by naming all that arises within them in her sensory world.

> In the first pool I enter the space and keep walk-
> ing around it. In the second pool I am at the bowl
> on the floor—more rocking—and in the third
> pool I'm still at the bowl, but here I experience
> a lot of sensations that maybe I would like to try
> to name.

> Back to the first pool: I kneel on the edge of the
> warm carpet and look back at you. I notice the
> color of your eyes. I close my eyes, stand, and walk
> into the space. I hear the doves outside, cooing.
> The floor is cold to my bare feet. I just keep
> walking around counterclockwise. I need to walk.
> I wonder now if needing is a sensation or an
> emotion for me.

> I teeter to my right and to my left, trying to find

some balance with my eyes closed. I am cold all over and wrap my shawl tightly around my shoulders. I experience the softness of my shawl, especially around my neck. Cold. I am cold. The first pool is about walking and being cold.

The second pool: This time, I don't pass by the bowl. I stop. The doves outside are quiet as I pull my shawl off and hold it in my right hand. I hear it land softly on the floor. Facing back into the room, I drop my right shoulder down to the floor. I am soft here and sensual. I am sinking. I come down to the floor on my knees, bending over into a crouched position. I begin to rock forward and back, forward and back, forward and back. I hear my exhale getting louder and louder as I bang back down onto my heels. I feel my out breath actually warming my chest under my chin. I rock and I rock as my whole body becomes warm again. The stone bowl beside me is always cool but I am becoming hot.

The third pool begins when my rocking ends. I can't remember how I curl onto my right side. I remember now getting a whiff of the lilacs just outside this end of the long wall of windows. Maybe it is in the same moment that I see a brief image of a baby in some kind of crib. I feel sensations of hunger. I feel pressure from my thumb on my cheek near my mouth.

I open my eyes and arrive into that subliminal

space and time that exists between moving and
coming out of moving, into this time and this
space. I look at you from this position on the
floor. As our eyes meet my belly contracts. I can
still feel this a little bit now as we are talking.
Lying there, the lilac smell, the baby image, my
thumb, our eye contact, an unease . . . maybe that's
an emotion? Here my nerves are not still—they
are buzzing. That's the last pool.

This mover no longer walks through the movement sequence while finding language for her work. As I listen to her speak on her cushion I notice
her hands moving in full synchrony with her words, as if shaping, clarifying
each one. Sometimes she speaks with her eyes open, sometimes she closes
them in an effort to stay closer to her experience. Now I offer witnessing.

At the beginning of your first pool I, too, hear the doves
cooing outside as my eyes meet yours here inside. You
walk onto the wooden floor and I see your eyelids close
in profile. As I see you wrap yourself in your shawl I am
cold and reach behind me for my own, pulling it around
my shoulders. Just as you arrive at the bowl and I see the
heel of your right foot lift into your last step. I hear one
dove loudly flap her wings as she takes off into flight.

Now at the bowl, your second pool, I see you drop your
shawl. I see it falling as if in slow motion. I also notice
the absence of the doves' cooing. Time slows down. I am
turning inward. You turn, facing the room, and come
down to the floor on all fours. I see you rock forward
and back, your toes tucked under your feet. I see you

*rock and rock and rock. I sense, softly see, the form of a
very small child, perhaps a baby.*

*After you rock—before you curl onto your right side—I
remember seeing you lie on your back. It is here that I
am acutely aware of a silence in the room as I see your
left arm lift straight up, your wrist extended. It pushes
upward, over the curve of the bowl. I see your hand suspended, suspended over the emptiness. Now I see your
wrist suddenly thrust upward and pull your arm back
down to your side.*

Yes. I forgot this. It is as though my arm is being
lifted, being moved. And my wrist is hot, full of
tiny vibrations. I cannot describe this very well. . . .
There is all time, all space, suddenly in this
moment. I am whole here.

*Yes, I deeply understand the difficulty in finding ways to
speak such an experience. Soon I see your legs curl up
as you roll to your right side, your thumb near your
mouth, and I remember my image of the baby. I'm
aware of my head tilting to the left so that I am seeing
you on the same visual plane that you see me when
you open your eyes.*

◖ Concentration requires rigor in the mover's practice. Trying to remember to stay present, to witness one's movement and to notice more and
more what accompanies it, is challenging work. Increased verbal articulation of a gesture, such as rocking, is what releases the mover from being

unconsciously merged with her experience. "Where are my hands, how are they placed on the floor, are my fingers splayed, is my head hanging down or tilted back, what is the quality of my sounding or breath, is my spine arched or straight?" In such a process the mover's inner witness is developing a dialogic relationship with her moving self. She sees herself moving and notices her inner experience in relationship to what her body is doing.

Increased verbal articulation of the sequence of a gesture series also develops. Though movement can be similar and different each time the mover works, here in the early study of the mover's and witness's experiences I am choosing to address the same basic sequence of movements repeatedly so that it becomes evident how each gesture expands in the moving body and in the developing consciousness. No movement exists in isolation. Each aspect of a series of gestures is equally important, especially if the movement is becoming a pattern, such as this woman's rocking. Dropping her shawl to the floor and following it down precedes the rocking. Lying on her side and experiencing her hand being dipped into the emptiness of the bowl follows the rocking.

Articulating the evolution of this series of gestures into the forming of pools is also clarifying. The pools are interdependent, each one necessary in relationship to the others. Sometimes movement in the earlier pools can feel like a warming up, a discharge of peripheral energy or a preparation. Such beginnings can be followed by a deepening of concentration, reflecting a shift in commitment toward a fuller presence of the inner witness. This can be followed by a wider focus in which movement slows down or resolves in relationship to what has just happened, a place for return and rest. With help from the witness, it is often only after the mover names the sequential pools within one session, or sometimes within a series of sessions, that meaningful relationship among them exists.

The witness can help the mover organize her mapping of her experiences by deepening her listening to her own experience in the presence of the mover. She can not only help to clarify places of question for the mover, as I do when this mover says she cannot remember how she arrived into a curled position on her side, but she can articulate and refine her own awareness of the arrival into and out of these shapes of the body moving in her presence, strengthening her own awareness practice.

As the relationship between the mover and the outer witness develops, the relationship within the mover, between her moving self and her inner witness, develops. She descends with increasing presence as unresolved or unconscious phenomena become known, felt in her body. These truths were often not safely witnessed during childhood or in primary adult relationships, thus leaving them unavailable for integration into the development of consciousness.

The mover's awareness of her outer witness becomes heightened as her work deepens into her sensory world. She begins to experience the witness as an inherent part of her process. She is opening into relationship to her witness as she opens to her experience of the phenomenal and natural complexities of projection, judgment, and interpretation regarding the presence and words of her witness. The mover can experience the witness as a parent, sibling, spouse, or friend in a positive or negative way.

A mover's awareness of how much literal space feels necessary, safe, or correct between herself and her witness can become essential to her process. There are times when the mover chooses to move closer to or farther away from her witness. The mover can ask the witness to move closer or farther away. The mover and the witness can discover together if touch is appropriate or comfortable. Slowly and over time the mover and the witness develop a vessel that could be understood as the relationship itself, holding all of what can be seen and what cannot be seen within the mover's work, within the witness's work, and within the relationship between the two.

One mystery that becomes apparent in this way of working is the experience of "being moved." Such a mysterious sensation can sometimes be understood as a precursor to energetic phenomena, or as the phenomena itself. Energetic phenomenon creates a transpersonal experience, one that is not sourced in personality, which could be understood as a combination of genetic coding and personal history. This mover realizes that she experiences an absence of the density of her personality when her moving self and her inner witness are one, as her hand is being dipped into the emptiness of the stone bowl: "There is all time, all space, suddenly in this moment. I am whole here." Different from the rest of her experiences, in which her inner witness is either merged with a sensation or in dialogue with it, here her inner witness is fully present and in direct experience, in a unitive state with her moving self.

Though she forgets about this moment, or perhaps chooses not to name it, I name it for two reasons. It is a physical movement, part of the map we are creating. I also speak it because I honor this movement as much as I honor all of her other movements in the gesture sequence. Sometimes movers do not speak of experiences like this one, experiences of energetic phenomena, as they are not sure if it is acceptable or believable by others. Often they themselves doubt such experiences. Doubt challenges the wish to share an already ineffable experience.

Spiritual growth, like physical and emotional growth, is developmental. At this time in this mover's practice, the primary intention is to ground and strengthen her inner witness. In doing so we are not only developing an appropriate and safe enough vessel that can hold conscious embodiment of unresolved aspects of personal history, but one that can hold transpersonal experiences as well. The presence of a healthy enough inner witness is a prerequisite for a safe reception of the full blessings of energetic phenomena. Experience of the mysteries can only be in service of the development of consciousness when they are embodied, when the mover's inner witness is aware of her physical movement and any accompanying inner phenomena.

The wind suddenly moves the branches of the persimmon and apple trees just beyond us in the orchard as I greet the mover on the small deck outside the studio doors. She sits on the bench, taking off her shoes, acknowledging one hawk circling above us. Now coming inside, we sit quietly together at the low table, preparing for the work.

> Today when you return from moving, briefly ground your work by naming the physical movement in sequential pools, naming accompanying sensation as you wish, and finally speak your experiences of emotions. This next step invites you toward a still fuller awareness of your inner life. If you don't return before, I will call you back in fifteen minutes.

Aware of the empty space, of not knowing what will happen and of trusting our relationship and this form to hold whatever emerges, I see the mover turning back to her left. She looks at me and then, turning a little more, she looks at the plant on the window seat, the red leaves infused with sunlight. Turning back the other way to her right, she now looks behind her at the lamp, the clock, and the small stone sculpture of a woman wrapping into herself on my desk. Now she looks at the pillows on the floor to the right of her feet, now across the room and up to the little window high above the stone bowl. I see her gazing a long time at this window of light before she closes her eyes.

Her inner witness:

> I long to be seen
> as I am
> all of me.

I am afraid
to be seen
all of me
in my shadow
in my light.

I fear my own
craziness
chaos.
I fear an explosion
of rage.
I fear the depths
of my pain
my despair.

I am afraid
of feeling it all
and I am afraid
of you seeing me
opening
to my own angst.

More often now
I arrive
at an inner edge
knowing I am close
to something I must know
but I cannot stay.

Just before I call the mover back, she opens her eyes and engages in extended eye contact from her position on her side in front of the bowl. Returning to her cushion, she begins to speak.

The first pool is anxiety. The second pool is frustration and fear when I'm at the bowl as scrubbing becomes pounding, then rocking. The third pool is when I lie on my side and feel comfort in eye contact, in my inner connection with you.

Now I'll go back and fill in. I look back at you, feeling so much uneasiness as I close my eyes. I hurl myself into the space, my head dropping toward my chest, pulling me into the emptiness. Half running, half hop-jumping, I fall this way and that into the space around me. I'm aware of missing the sound of the doves. I stop abruptly near the bowl, take three steps toward it with my eyes barely open, and wrap my shawl tightly around myself, not because I am cold but because I am anxious. Standing here I suddenly lift up my head, open my eyes, and turn to look at you for a brief second. Now closing my eyes, my head falls back down, down into my covering, down into my doubt, doubting myself, doubting this work.

Unwrapping, I drop my shawl to the floor near the bowl, exhaling really loudly. When I hear the shawl land I get down on my hands and knees, grab the shawl and start scrubbing the floor with it. Clean. Preparing. I make this space clean.

Scrubbing turns into pounding. I am tense in my arms and hands. As I pound the floor I yell. Feeling impatient, sick of myself, I yell, I rock. I have the whole room to move in, to do anything

I want and all I do is the same thing over and over, rocking, rocking, rocking. I am appalled by my captivity, by the tyranny of this movement.

Suddenly, for a brief second, I am all one being, no awareness of separate parts or specific sensation. I am a terrified rocking baby, pressing my wrists into the floor, banging back down onto my heels. I stop.

On my side again, I open my eyes before you call time because I need to see your eyes. I lie there on my side, my back to the bowl, looking for you, looking for me. As our eyes meet I am surprised by a sudden rush of feeling, of needing to crawl into your lap. I begin to consider this desire, and my mind floods with logistics, like how would I ever cross the space and is it allowed and what would I do if I were in your lap. Slowly I realize the time for such a leap is past and I am simply lying here at the bowl, staring into your eyes, relaxing, feeling comforted.

As the mover speaks, as I listen, I feel a warmth within, a warmth between us, as we again, in this moment, look so clearly into each other's eyes. I offer witnessing.

As you close your eyes and hurl yourself into the space, headfirst, I am washed again in gratitude to you for trusting me to witness you here, in this practice.

You take three steps toward the bowl and seeing the soles of your feet, one by one, I am vulnerable. As I see

you standing, looking into my eyes, I am trusting.
Hearing you exhale, I am relieved. I see you drop your
shawl, then yourself, down to the floor and now I hear
you yell. I hear you. I hear you still yelling, feeling your
yelling sounds thumping inside my belly. I see you scrub.
My belly contracts. I see you rock and rock and rock,
pressing your wrists, pressing them into the floor. I see a
baby rocking.

My vision narrows toward seeing you as very small,
sensing there is no one near you. You fill the space. I feel
hope as I see you safely here, moving into that which
has been calling. I am not afraid. I trust your inner wit-
ness to guide you safely. When you open your eyes,
curled on your side, and you look at me, I am full of
tenderness, as if I am holding you.

◻ This mover is learning to choose to surrender or not surrender to an
impulse. Once descending, sometimes she can choose to stay a little longer.
Such decisions are often made intuitively. As movers identify physical
movement, sensation, emotion, and thought with more acuity, awareness of
intuitive experience often surfaces, becoming more of an active guide. She
learns to honor her impatience with repeated impulse, to honor her fear,
and eventually she learns to honor her intuitive sense that it is time to commit to a fuller embodiment of this gestalt because she must. What else is
there to do?

The witness can model experiences of intuitive knowing, as I did in this
round in the third pool when I speak about not sensing or seeing anyone
near the mover, experiencing a change in my spatial perception: *"You fill the
space."* Within this process we are both listening more and more carefully
to the subtleties of verbal expression in order to know more clearly what

our experiences actually are. We are discerning physical movement from sensation, sensation from emotion, memory from thought, thought from intuition. We are sorting, separating each moment from another moment, each gesture from another, each word, each longing, each fear. We are trusting in an inevitable discovery of an inherent order, an inherent wholeness.

Stumbling into language that comes directly from embodiment encourages change from old ways of speaking. This is because habit, sometimes wisely, sometimes infuriatingly, tenaciously keeps us at varying distances from our experience. For a mover there is significant difference between: my story is about being a baby, I imagine I am a baby, I'm thinking of a baby, I feel like a baby, I must look like a baby, and "I am a baby." For a witness there is great difference between *"I imagine a baby is rocking"* and *"I see a baby rocking."* Imagination can begin in the conceptual world. As images move down and into embodiment, toward becoming directly known, the experience of self as one has known it is altered. Such distinctions deserve discernment, deserve words that move closer to the subjective truth. A call toward impeccability becomes apparent. A call toward translating this way of speaking with consciousness into daily life becomes urgently clear.

At this time in this process, the mover often manifests an increasing need to report everything that happens, the detail of every gesture, when it happens, where it happens in the room, what she feels, thinks, knows. It is as if there is an audible plea from within each moment, waiting to be known, to be named. When this occurs it is essential that the witness acknowledge such longing by listening and attending to the detail that is being marked with such thoughtfulness by the mover. This constant attention to detail by both mover and witness supports a strengthening of the dialogic relationship that the mover is developing, not only between herself and her outer witness but between her moving self and her inner witness.

Naming detail unveils the natural occurrence of repetition, a central force within the body's wisdom, a phenomenon necessary for growth.

Though new movements appear throughout these series of sessions, movement patterns are increasingly repeated. The repetition of the patterns themselves—"all I do is the same thing over and over"—as well as repetitive movements within each pattern—"rocking, rocking, rocking"—reflect experience buried in the tissues. Webbed into the nervous system in early life, these patterns, unconsciously created for excellent reasons, become habit. In the course of development they become less and less useful and eventually interfere with an ability to live well in the present.

The witness/teacher guides the mover toward reflecting repetition of movement in her speech patterns as she concisely repeats specific phrases to emphasize her own experience as witness—*"I hear you yell. I hear you. I hear you still yelling."* Cadence, inflection, tone, deeply important in the moving experience itself, can infuse the experience of speech with more clarity, with more truth.

We continue to meet. Today the morning fog is visibly tumbling in from the sea, filling the hills and the valleys around us. I feel warmly wrapped in it as I light a candle and greet the mover. She arrives a bit late, wrapped in her white shawl, stating that she wants to move immediately. Before she moves I remind her that, as the length of her moving time is increasing, it is she who decides when to end. However, depending on the clock, I will call her back at a certain time if she is still moving so that there is sufficient time to dialogue about our experiences. Now she rushes into the emptiness, running, circling the space. Stopping suddenly, she makes eye contact with me, walks toward the bowl, and closes her eyes.

Her inner witness:

> I long
> to be
> unconditionally loved.
> I am afraid
> of this longing
> because I am unworthy.
>
> I crave the light
> and endlessly arrive
> into the darkness
> of my own being.
> I lose track of time
> when I move.
> Powerful experiences
> occur and yet
> I have
> no adequate words
> afterward.
>
> I don't know.
> I don't know.

Twenty minutes have passed. I call her name and tell her it is time to bring her experience to an end, reminding her to take as much time as she needs for making the transition back. When she is ready, she speaks.

> Except at the very end, there is only one pool
> the entire time—fear. I know it now as a specific

sensation inside my heart, like a run of quick, painful jabs of a needle. And I know it in my belly, way down, a miserable shredding within a gaping emptiness. I am afraid even before I close my eyes. I run in with my body stiff, my chin pulled into my neck, my shoulders pulled up and tense. Stopping short, I walk to the bowl. I see your eyes. I close mine. My face feels tight. My breathing is heavy. I drop my shawl to the floor, follow it as if I am entering another world. On my hands and knees, my wrists press hard into the floor. With my back arched I rock backward onto my heels and now forward toward that pressing place, my wrists pressing, held down, tied down. Rocking and rocking, rocking and rocking, I repeat this same exact movement, so exactly the same that now I know the instant I am not doing it "right."

Space and time vanish around me as I am locked into this particular sensation, an elongated, narrow, and perilous place that I totally fill. I am only nerve endings. There is nothing else in my knowing. I am only this. Now screaming, I am rocking. Rocking, I am screaming. Here I am. Here I am.

A terror sears through me right before I know, directly know in my body, that I am surrendering. Within the fear of the unknown, yet knowing you are here, it's as if I descend in spite of the terror, feeling as though I am risking my life. I surrender in this moment and allow myself to actually

become the baby abandoned, the baby tied down,
starving for food. I am the baby in the hospital.
I know the slats of the crib. I am screaming for
Mama. I call to her. I call and call to her until
I drop with exhaustion. When I open my eyes you
are here, sitting near me by the bowl. Thank you.
I need your presence close in. I am spent, relieved.

Telling you this now, I feel a tiny shaking in my
legs, my stomach, my arms and hands, my jaw.
I seem to be shivering all over but I am not cold.
Something's gone. I can feel a new empty space
inside.

Sitting on the floor here next to the mover, I am aware that I am also spent
and deeply relieved. I speak, full of love and gratitude.

*I see you rocking and rocking and rocking. I hear you
calling and calling. I am moved into and through a narrow passage as I see you, as I see a baby, opening to the
fullness of terror in the moment of abandonment. I get
up and come toward you because I want to be near you.
I trust you, your timing, your presence. I love this baby.*

There are times, though rare, when as a witness I intuitively choose to
go nearer to a mover, my presence bringing the space around her into a
smaller circle, more contained, more personal. Here I go to her for these
reasons and to simply be with another who is suffering so.

A mover can work with original trauma in the discipline of Authentic
Movement because of a developing inner witness in relationship to the
presence of an outer witness. Trauma occurs in the nervous system. It is the

body's direct experience of shock that threatens physical and/or psychological integrity, creating an experience of total helplessness. If the trauma occurs in infancy or early childhood, there is no inner witness and therefore no way of remembering the occurrence without work based in body awareness.

If the person is old enough when the trauma occurs to have some experience of an inner witness, usually the inner witness is not able to remain in a conscious relationship to the trauma because of experiencing overwhelm and shock. The inner witness escapes or evaporates for clear reasons—for survival. The body knows, remembers trauma at a cellular level, but without a present and strong enough inner witness when the trauma is occurring, what the body knows cannot be remembered. The experience of the inner witness and the experience of the body can be severed. When this happens, sometimes for some people, the body can become a threat, a container of unconscious, unexpressed darkness and terror.

Because of its intimacy and safety, the dyadic format in the discipline of Authentic Movement is an excellent one for individuals, like this mover, who suffer from trauma. Because infant development is totally enmeshed in the relationship or absence of relationship with a nurturing figure, when reentering such material later only one other person, one witness, is necessary. A group with other movers and many witnesses may be too overwhelming, not only for the mover but for others in the group.

Knowledge of developmental movement and psychology importantly informs a witness's ability to see at what phase of development the mover is working. I could see that this mover's gestures and sounds were associated with the first eighteen months of life: her thumb repeatedly near her mouth, her persistent rocking, the way in which she rocked back onto her heels, the arch of her back, the quality of her cries. In this situation the mover becomes aware of her thumb near her mouth, her rocking, and an image of a baby. It becomes apparent to us both that, as the quality of affect evolves within these movements, she is working in a preverbal time.

Two intimately interrelated realities are essential for previously bound and embedded trauma to safely emerge into consciousness: a strong enough inner witness and a compassionate and strong enough outer witness. If both aspects are not present, reentering the horrific experience of sensations and emotions can retraumatize the individual. A strong enough inner witness means that the person can track her movements and inner experiences while immersed in them. Her inner witness also must be able to modulate her movement experience. She must learn, with help from her witness, how to soothe or calm herself, to not allow herself to become overwhelmed by too much feeling too quickly.

Such strengthening of her inner witness occurs only in direct relationship to the presence of a good enough outer witness. When suffering occurs in the original trauma, staying in relationship to the other is usually not possible because the other can often be another helpless victim or a helpless witness. When the pain is inflicted by another human being, staying in relationship to the utter darkness of that unconscious presence is most likely impossible. In this discipline the presence of another, the outer witness, can offer conscious witnessing that was absent during the original trauma.

The witness must be able to stay conscious in the presence of such deep suffering instead of merging with her mover's experience. She must be able to remain in her own separate, dialogic experience, which often can feel empathic, full of her own sensations and emotions. As this happens she learns to contain her own experiences in order to honor and protect her mover's boundaries and timing. In doing so she is opening toward her longing for an experience of a compassionate presence in relationship to suffering. Such presence can be experienced by the mover as the presence of one who desires to see the truth, who can bear to see the truth.

When the timing was correct for this mover she relived the original trauma, suffering abandonment again. The experience could no longer be denied, rearranged, or prevented. Often when a mover is working with the intensity of sensory and emotional energy related to personal history, the experience is that of arriving into a specific place with no space around it or outside of it. This mover says: "Space and time vanish around me as I choose to stay within this particular sensation, an elongated, narrow place which I totally fill."

Rather than changing the outcome, safely reentering her own truth is what can release the bound energy into emerging consciousness, creating a shift in the nervous system itself, creating healing. Wounds never heal completely, perhaps mysteriously protecting who we are becoming because of our experience of our past. In this way of work it is not necessary to try to find meaning in such monumental passages because spontaneous insight usually synchronistically occurs. Keeping track of experience, staying conscious of what is happening, automatically prepares and opens the psyche for a new way of knowing that appears inside the mover's relationship with herself, with her witness, and within natural, organic timing. Paradoxically, becoming more conscious—the new way of knowing—means letting go of an old way of knowing. Loss is inevitable. "Something's gone. I can feel a new empty space inside." Descending into and through a movement pattern intrinsically and thus automatically expands the movement repertoire.

As this mover experiences her outer witness's developing compassion, it becomes possible for her to experience her own suffering becoming compassion and then for her to bring a more compassionate presence in relationship to another. In the teaching practice, as the mover becomes more able to see and to accept herself as she is, she is preparing to experience the presence of another mover, to share the space with her in the presence of an outer witness.

The Moving Witness

Then our Lord said to her: "Place thy hands
against My hands, and thy feet against My feet,
and thy breast against My breast, and in such
wise shall be so much helped by thee that
My pain will be less."

LUKARDIS OF OBERWEIMAR

○ All that we learn about witness consciousness is sourced in the experience of being a mover. In the structure of the form, the natural bridge
between the mover and the witness is the moving witness. When the wit-
ness/teacher and two different movers agree that the inner witness is strong
enough within each of them, they move into the empty space at the same
time in the presence of the outer witness. They become each other's moving witness. Though each mover has her eyes closed the presence of the
other is palpable, making each a blind but vital witness for the other.

The possibility of relationship between these two movers enters the
consciousness of each mover. For each, the "other" is no longer just the witness, predictably sitting still and silent to the side of the movement space.
This "other" is right here, intending to listen more and more deeply within
herself while intending to maintain some kind of awareness of the other
mover in the same space.

Even though touch becomes inevitable between two movers in the same space, often sounds of another are the first felt signs of the actual presence of someone else. Sounds of the other mover can fill, invade, support, soothe, frighten, or disarm a mover. When sound happens a mover can either receive it, resist it by covering her ears or moving away from it, or she can embody her ambivalence by repeatedly moving toward and then away from it. Because it is virtually impossible to not hear a sound, whether experienced as positive or negative, each sound has a potential for significantly affecting the other mover's work.

Movers can intend to try to find each other to make physical contact or they can spontaneously discover contact. When touch happens a mover can choose to embody her wish to experience it or she can clearly refuse it by moving away. She can also embody her ambivalence by both moving away from the touch and then moving toward it. The practice of discernment here can enliven the work for each mover, whether the encounter is nourishing, a welcomed blessing, challenging, or disruptive. Certain moments of meeting another can become critical turning points in the mover's work.

Trust in each other's presence requires a commitment to open their eyes if either makes big, sudden, or fast movements in order to protect now not only themselves but the other mover. When two movers are on the floor at the same time they simply are in relationship to each other whether they hear or touch each other, whether they speak about it afterward or not. The subterranean connection becomes mysterious and compelling, creating a very particular bond between movers. At times it is as though what happens for each individual only happens because of the presence of the other mover.

It is here, early in the evolution of this form, that a mover directly bumps into a familiar and profoundly human challenge that will continue to deepen into this practice: the embodied tension between her longing to be in conscious relationship with herself and, simultaneously, her longing to be in conscious relationship with another.

In the late afternoon I greet the woman with the white shawl and another woman with long gray hair who has also had in-depth experience as a mover alone in my presence. Settling inside on the carpet near the low table, we begin in the first triad of the practice. After the movers make eye contact with each other and with me, the mover with the long hair lies down on her side on the carpet's edge, dangling her left hand into the space before she moves in.

Her inner witness:

> I protect myself
> with my hair
> wrapped around
> my face as I
> roll in
> wondering
> what this will be like
> with you here.
>
> I am not alone
> in this emptiness.
> I hear you.
> I sense your presence.
> I hear you
> breathing.
>
> This space feels
> so small

with nowhere
to hide
from myself
from my fears
of encountering you.

What will I do
if you touch me?
How do I
without words
let you know?

I don't want
to hurt your feelings.
I am terrified
of being touched
in this vulnerable
place
of blindness
of not knowing.

I am not ready.
I must do my own
work.

The mover with the white shawl steps backward into the space, her right foot straight out behind her, her toes turning inward, her heel landing suddenly, quickly onto the floor. I see her palms pressed together over her heart, her head dropped to her left side, her chin slightly tilted upward.

Her inner witness:

> I am not alone
> in this emptiness.
> I hear you.
> I sense your presence.
> I hear you
> breathing.
> I hear your body
> moving on the floor
> pausing
> now moving again.
>
> How do I tell you
> I want contact.
> You are round
> and soft
> an imagined comfort
> for my angles
> my sharp corners.
>
> Dare I reach out
> and try to
> find
> you?

The woman with the gray hair continues to roll, pulling her right knee up toward her face as she lands on her belly, then rolls onto her back and over to the other side, now pulling her left knee up.

Her inner witness:

> I imagine
> our witness prefers
> your buoyancy
> to my slow slumping
> here on the floor.
>
> Your movements
> are quick and direct.
> My lethargic roll
> feels even heavier
> in comparison.
> Your lithe body is the one
> for which I've always
> yearned.
>
> My body
> my round and full body
> challenges me
> challenges me
> every day
> of my life.

Now the movers work with their projections, not only onto me as the witness but onto each other as well. I see the woman with her white shawl tied tightly around her hips like a skirt, who has been walking backward in a circle, now walking backward toward the bowl. The woman with the gray hair rolls very slowly into the space behind her, into the other mover's legs. Rolling and now stopping, I hear her sighing and then she becomes very still.

Her inner witness:

> Here you are
> in my pool!
> and I am afraid.
> I don't want
> to hurt your feelings.
> I cannot do this.
> I cannot bear this.
> Don't touch me
> in this vulnerable
> place
> of blindness
> of not knowing.
>
> I am not ready.
> I must leave.
> I must leave.

The woman standing at the bowl stops moving. I can't even see that she is breathing. No part of her moves. I see tears falling from her eyes. She now slowly bends her knees and tentatively reaches her right hand down toward the other mover. Her fingers groping, they land on the mover's shoulder. She taps three times there, as the other mover rolls away into the emptiness. Standing alone and straightening her knees, she turns and walks straight ahead toward the bowl, another empty space.

Her inner witness:

> I want to stay
> but it is unbearable
> to even imagine

that I am
imposing.

You go away
and I remember
from somewhere
somehow
that gnaw
in my belly
twist and contract
being left
shockingly familiar.

Twenty minutes have passed and I say the names of the movers and ask them to bring their experiences to an end. I see the movers look at each other and then at me. Returning to their cushions here on the carpet, we begin speaking together.

As your ability strengthens to integrate what your bodies are doing, in what sequence the pools of movement are occurring and what accompanying sensations and emotions are felt, more opportunity for discernment arises. Within this growing clarity you can increasingly choose what gestures, what sensations, what emotions you want to speak in more detail, and what is not necessary to speak, perhaps because speaking it might be premature or maybe it has already been integrated.

Each mover, with eyes open, briefly names her pools, shaped especially by the physical movement, offering a simple map for each other and for me as the witness. Now the movers each choose one place they want to enter more fully. This time, as is often the case with two movers, they first choose to dialogue about their experience of an encounter. I listen. Now I choose

witnessing for each mover that is in response to work she has spoken. I
speak first to the woman with the gray hair.

> *I see you rolling into the space. Each time as you roll
> onto your belly, your body flat on the oak wood floor,
> your knee coming up toward your face, I am satisfied,
> grounded, feeling my whole body as one form. Yes, as
> you roll into the legs of the other mover, I am sus-
> pended, not knowing what is going to happen.*

I speak to the woman with the white shawl.

> *I see you stepping backward into the space. As your
> head drops to the side your shoulders and upper torso
> follow until you are turning backward into a spiraling
> circle, your feet stepping down toe heel, toe heel. I am
> invited toward a center place that is somehow always
> behind you. I am eager and ready to go there with you.*

I continue speaking to the woman with the white shawl, addressing the
moment of touch.

> *As you bend to touch the other mover who appears
> behind you I want you to have the opportunity to sus-
> tain this experience of touch for as long as you wish. I
> feel warmth in my chest.*

Now, concerning the same moment, I speak to the woman with the long
gray hair.

> *And as you are touched, my eyes widen. I don't want
> you to stay in this moment of touch any longer than
> you choose. It is right here that I remember that this*

work is not about seeking pleasure and avoiding pain. It is about discovering, accepting, enduring our own truth and the truth of the other.

The season is dry, the daisies are abundant, pushing up tall and white around the bowl of water at the corner of the deck. Dusk slips into their exuberance, into the studio. The two women arrive again, after months of work here together. I light a candle and we begin by making eye contact with each other. Now the movers stand at the carpet's edge and step in.

As always when witnessing more than one person, I find myself not only witnessing each one but also witnessing my own experience of relationship between the two. What is the connection? I am looking at this one, now looking at that one, now the space in between. Light, shapes, and qualities of energy create a third essence quickly forming in my presence. May I be able to stay in conscious relationship to all that arises within each mover and simultaneously to all that arises within their relationship.

The space is filled for twenty-five minutes with the movement of these two women and now the space is emptied as I call their names, asking them to bring their experiences to an end. They make eye contact with each other and then with me and return to their cushions. Both movers name their pools sequentially and then choose to speak in more detail about the beginning and middle pools of their work. The woman with the long gray hair speaks first.

I walk straight in and to my left, over toward the
wall with all of the windows. Turning, I walk
across to the other wall and turning again, back
across the room. I am pacing, sighing, my hands
flailing at my sides. Over here, back across to
there, this way, that way, I am frustrated, agitated.
Pacing, I don't know where to go, what to do.

Now the woman with the white shawl speaks.

I step in, placing the outside edge of my thumb
on the top of my head, my fingers stretched open
and upward. With my hand staying wide, my
thumb presses down onto my forehead, now following the ridge of my nose, across the midline of
my lips and my chin, and now marking the middle of my torso. Walking slowly, carving this line,
I'm splitting my chest in two. Without understanding, without meaning, I need to do this. This
gesture is correct. Over and over my thumb trav-
erses this pathway until my whole body follows
and I sit down. My legs are crossed.

My hand pulls my arm straight out in front of me.
My wrist pushes, flexes, and my palm faces away. I
am waiting. I am waiting. Outer movement stops
and I become only my hand, listening. My belly
begins to shake. Water flows from my eyes. My
head moves from side to side, side to side. "No." I
whisper "no" as small cries escape from my mouth.

The woman with the gray hair continues.

> I hear the other mover's whispers, her small cries,
> her inhales fast and quick. I hear her crying.
> I hear her cries, her whispers, her cries. Back and
> forth, back and forth, and my heart breaks open
> and I am only my desire to come to her. No
> thoughts, no big decision. I simply come. I sit
> behind her. We are back to back, back of heart
> to back of heart. Love moves.

The woman with the white shawl responds.

> As darkness is pushed out through my hand, I
> receive the light of your presence fillling my back,
> my front, now all of me.

I offer witnessing to each mover specifically in relationship to what they
have shared and now I offer witnessing of my experience of their moving
relationship. First I address the woman with the white shawl.

> *I see you sitting in the center of the room,*
> *your legs crossed, your thumb now leaving*
> *your body and stretching into the space in*
> *front of you, stopping, your palm facing out.*

Turning slightly, I speak to the woman with the long gray hair.

> *I see you pacing the floor, over there, over*
> *here, pacing, flailing.*

Continuing, I address both women.

*Anticipation rises, a prickly sensation in my
shoulders and arms, in my throat, in my
jaw. The space between the two of you
becomes charged, scarlet and electric. I focus
there. And now, without knowing how this
happens, I see you back to back and the
color of compassion floods my heart. I am
opened.*

The movers continue to speak more moments in their moving experience
and receive more witnessing until it is time to leave. They walk out into an
early, quiet darkness created by the fog. Saying good-bye at the door I can
smell the freshness of the lavender growing here nearby, a comforting fra-
grance, a salve for the senses.

Time passes. Here come these two women, arriving together on the path
just as the doves fly into their house for the night. Here come the two dogs,
greeting the two women who are greeting the birds. The movers leave their
bags and shawls on the window seat just inside the door to their right and
it is time to begin. The woman whose gray hair is today on top of her head
names the intense pain in her right shoulder. We all make eye contact and
the women stand at the edge of the space once again, move for forty minutes and return, making eye contact one more time.

Drinking hot tea, the two women mark their pools of movements and then begin to dialogue, the woman with the gray hair speaking first, followed by the woman with the white shawl.

> My pain is gone. What happened? I begin by immediately lying on my back on the floor, I think in the center of the room. My arms are bent over my torso, my hands limp, facing my chest, my wrists tingling. I am so vulnerable, small, and also annoyed, not wanting to be bothered with this pain here now in this practice.

> > I begin standing over by the bowl, swinging my right arm full out in front of me, chanting a little sound with good spirit. This swinging of one arm leads me into the space, galloping around in a circle, facing out. I think you are inside this circle. My chanting gets louder and I feel exuberant.

> My right hand is trembling, trembling and I hear you near me, but oddly, I don't feel afraid. I am deep inside, holding this pain, this persistent pre-occupation.

> > My chanting dance brings me onto all fours, my head hanging down. My hands and feet move in a rhythm. I am touching the floor here and there and suddenly here I am also touching your leg.

I feel your hand on my leg just as I am sitting up,
my hands still in front of my chest, my palms facing in, my head down. I welcome your touch. I
reach out and touch your hair with my finger and
my thumb. Soon my head slides very slowly into
this side of your neck. This is a soft place. I am
safe. Oh, you hold me here. I feel your hand
strong and firm on my back. I can meet you here.

> Yes, I am so grateful for this connection
> with you, these sounds chanting quietly
> inside my head, these rhythms in my
> feet, my torso, my hands. My right hand
> taps them with love on your back.

I am so happy here, imbibing your rhythms as
they invisibly invite me to move. I realize only
now in speaking that as my movement becomes
authentic my relationship to my pain changes. I
actually forgot about my shoulder.

> Yes I also forgot about it. Here at the
> end, as we're helping each other up, I
> feel playful, prancing these rhythms
> with delight. You become my sister and
> I am again safe with her, dancing and
> laughing in our secret happy place, our
> escape place from our parents' pain.
> Thank you, thank you.

When movers are so clear and able to witness themselves and each other,
external witnessing can be redundant. Here I have nothing to offer in this
rich dialogue except naming my gratitude for the privilege of witnessing.

⧠ Movers are encouraged to name places of physical pain or vulnerability in support of feeling safe when they enter the movement floor with others who have their eyes closed. In general the mover is invited to enter the space with no agenda, with no specific plans regarding personal-history work, current challenging situations, or an intention to create spiritual experience. Can she enter the emptiness not knowing, not knowing what will arise within herself, within the other, within their relationship?

When the inner witness of a mover is strong and loving enough, the longing to see another guides her into becoming an outer witness of another mover. It is as though instead of moving with the other mover she shifts to the side of the movement space, opens her eyes, and now witnesses the other mover working with her eyes closed. She approaches witness practice with the same three questions: can she sit in the presence of a mover not knowing what will arise within herself, within her mover, and within their relationship?

Developing
Witness
Consciousness

Self-revelation requires encounter
between self and other:
the revealer needs an other
to whom to be revealed.

RABBI ARTHUR GREEN

The Witness

How
Do I
Listen to others?
As if everyone were my Master
Speaking to me
His
Cherished
Last
Words.

HAFIZ

From moving witness to witness, from sensing a mover with eyes closed to seeing a mover with eyes open, each individual enters the next place of practice and study within the development of embodied consciousness. The mover chooses to become a witness.

The witness's experience is completely dependent on the presence of the mover, who is the primary catalyst for all that stirs within her. The mover's experience is completely dependent on the presence of the witness. The precious relationship between the mover and the witness is the ground form of the practice. It is this dyadic relationship, both conscious and unconscious, which holds, as if it were a bowl like the one carved in stone here in the studio, the contents and processes that arise, resonate, and evaporate within it.

This relationship frees each member to embrace a half of the whole of the mover/witness dynamic. There is the one who moves with eyes closed, expressing experience, and there is the one who is still, with eyes open, containing experience. Here the discipline balances opposing forces, each potentially becoming the other, each a necessary element of practice toward presence. The bridge between the forces of mover and witness consciousness is the inner witness.

Who is the witness? There are two separate but intimately related centers in the development of witness consciousness. One, which is intrapersonal, concerns the developing inner witness, the continuing desire from the moving practice to see oneself more clearly. The witness does not look at or observe her mover, bringing her focus solely over there, onto the moving body. Instead the witness is participating, opening to the complexities of her own experience from moment to moment, here within her own being, in the presence of the mover. The other center, which is interpersonal, concerns the desire to see another more clearly, to be in service to the mover, which is what brings the witness into the presence of a mover.

The witness's inner witness continues to develop within the primary work of tracking. She begins as she began in her moving practice, by tracking physical movement. Though the new witness has prepared for this experience of tracking physical movement in her work as a mover, tracking her own movement with her eyes closed is different than tracking another's movement with her eyes open. For some new witnesses, remembering the physical movements and their sequence can be difficult because the movements are not being directly recorded in the body when witnessing, as they are when moving. For others for whom the visual field is a dominant one, remembering can be supported by open eyes, making consciousness more available.

Once the shared intention of mover and witness shifts to include more than just the mover's physical expression, the tasks of the witness multiply. The mover contains and expresses her own experience, tracking it as it occurs. While the witness contains her own experience, not expressing it through movement, she also at the same time is tracking what her mover is doing and simultaneously tracking her own inner experience in response.

"Where am I? What am I doing now? Here I am, seeing you pacing the floor, over there, over here, pacing, flailing." The outer witness was first a beginning mover, learning the practice of tracking from her outer witness. Now she teaches her mover about tracking. She becomes a model for the development of the mover's inner witness, the aspect of the mover which is becoming conscious of her own experience, her own truth.

Because a phenomenal relationship exists between truth and beauty, as the witness opens toward her own truth she can find it to be inextricably bound to her own experience of aesthetics. While concentrating on the mover's work, especially when a mover is visibly focused inward, the witness can be seized or soothed, awed or changed by a sudden awareness of the incomprehensible presence, the force of beauty itself.

Her inner witness:

> *I see the late afternoon light falling onto your body.*
> *Silence expands as I see you stand on one leg, your other leg*
> *lifted high behind you. I see the rippling sleeves of your blouse,*
> *shining and black, as your hand reaches to hold onto the window*
> *frame. I see the palm of your other hand, fingers shaped,*
> *extended in the air, as your torso bends back, your hair falling*
> *into a column of sunlight. Your white pants, wide at the bottom,*
> *flutter as you subtly work to maintain balance. Nourished,*
> *renewed, I see you. I know beauty.*

In the development of witness consciousness the witness learns to see as she studies her experience of merging with her mover, of being in dialogic relationship with her mover and, in moments of grace, experiencing the blessing of a unitive state with her mover. In this process what matters is the seeing, seeing what is here in this moment within and without. The word *seeing* is used to describe literally a seeing and also a listening, an intuitive sensing.

As the longing to see clearly is placed into a witness practice, the discovery of the countless internal obstacles to such a desire inevitably occurs. Now the witness commits to her longing as she begins a sustained and extensive exploration of the unknown.

Her inner witness:

> *I long to open*
> *to surrender*
> *to my own experience*
> *because of your*
> *presence*
> *your trust.*
>
> *I wish to see*
> *you clearly*
> *and I fear*
> *my own density*
> *will interfere.*
>
> *I am embarrassed*
> *about the business*
> *of my mind.*
> *I don't want to judge you*
> *or project my own experience*
> *onto you.*
> *May I be able*
> *to honor the mysteries*
> *of your being.*
> *It is the grace*
> *of clear, silent awareness*
> *for which I long.*

The Silent Witness

The monk is "trying to understand" when in fact he ought to try to look. The mysterious and cryptic sayings of Zen become much simpler when we see them in the whole context of Buddhist "mindfulness" or awareness, which in its most elementary form consists in that "bare attention," which simply sees what is right there and does not add any comment, any interpretation, any judgment, any conclusion. It just sees.

D. T. SUZUKI

Because conscious speaking requires study and practice, before a person honors the privilege of speaking to a mover she commits to the silent witness practice. The silence protects the witness from premature responsibility and the mover from the possibility of receiving unconscious witnessing.

The silent witness studies the workings of her own mind in a concentrated way. First she has an opportunity to notice how she transfers her ability to track her own experience as a mover to tracking another person's movements. Next she practices tracking the mover's physical movement in relationship to her own accompanying experience of sensation, emotion, and thought. Once comfortable with this work she adds her awareness of how she opens to the content of her inner experiences as a witness. Often in the beginning she can feel flooded with judgments, projections, and interpretations. Such experiences, natural and dynamic forces of being human, become gifts, vital invitations for attention by her conscious mind. It is here in the evolution of the discipline that specific space is made for direct and generous attention to such phenomena.

The shape of the silent witness practice is the second triad: a speaking witness, a silent witness, and a mover. The opportunity for the silent witness to witness a mover and a speaking witness working together is invaluable. The mover can feel supported by the presence of the silent witness and at the same time feel safely held by the experienced speaking witness. Every hour of working as a silent witness invites another hour of supervision with the teacher, the speaking witness. It is within this frame that the silent witness can safely give voice to her experience. The supervision work can occur individually or in a group format with others who are committed to a silent witness practice.

In the discipline of Authentic Movement it is the other, the mover, who stimulates rich, unique, and often challenging material for the witness to behold. What matters more than the specific content experienced within the witness, though she must address it, is how she comes into relationship to it. The silent witness can learn how to bring her awareness to such experiences, thus learning about her own nature, her personality, and her longing toward presence.

The woman with her white shawl tucked in her bag approaches the deck, sending a wild bird fleeing from his bath in the bowl of water across from the bench. Another woman, after giving tiny cookies to the dogs, arrives and sits on the bench, taking off her shoes. The lilac blooms. The windows are open. The stone bowl in the corner of the room is empty.

Inside, pulling up a third chair, I introduce the moving practice to the new mover, asking her to notice her physical movement and to gather it into pools of sequential development. As she prepares to move she makes eye contact with me, placing her black shawl loosely over her head and shoulders. I now see her looking at the silent witness for an extended moment and then walking to the carpet's edge. Facing the emptiness, she closes her eyes as she kneels, crossing her wrists and placing her palms flat on her chest. Now I see her crawl onto the floor.

I see the silent witness looking at the mover, her hands tightly holding the arms of the chair.

Her inner witness:

> *Oh no, you*
> *kneel and I*
> *feel like*
> *running away.*
> *You're praying*
> *I'm running*
> *I'm sorry*
> *I'm running away*
> *as I see you*
> *pray.*

I don't know how
to pray.
I can't do it.
I will never
find my God
never.

◖ The gifts from the mover to the witness are abundant, often less obvious compared to the gifts of presence that the witness can offer the mover. When the silent witness and I speak together later in supervision, she explores her intense feelings that occur as soon as the mover begins. As the mover kneels under her black shawl and crosses her hands on her chest, the silent witness sees a religious posture. She discovers feelings of anger, betrayal, and confusion sourced in her personal history. Under these feelings she receives a glimpse of her longing for an authentic communion with the Divine. There is space here for the silent witness to safely open to all that is arising within her. Such work introduces new questions about her own boundaries. Returning to her silent witness practice, she continues the studio work.

Her inner witness:

I see you
crawling
and you keep crawling
you keep crawling.
I become frightened
as you crawl.
My throat constricts.
You look frantic.
You are frantic.

◯ Here the silent witness explores her experience of judgment of her mover. Judgment often begins with a sense that the mover "looks" beautiful or ugly, happy or sad, calm or frantic. Judgment can be positive or negative. But such information is rarely helpful to the mover or the witness. If a witness feels that her mover is frantic, instead of the statement "you are frantic" or " you look frantic" or "my experience is that you are frantic," the question that the witness must ask herself is: "How do I feel in the presence of someone who I name as frantic?" She might feel exhausted, helpless, distressed, or sad. Next the witness listens to how the mover expresses her experience. If the mover speaks of her exhaustion while crawling and the witness has realized that indeed she feels exhausted, if she were a speaking witness it would be appropriate for her to share this with her mover. If the witness's emotional experience is clearly different from the mover's, it would be in the service of the mover for the speaking witness to contain her emotional response and only offer her tracking of the gestures. There is a critical difference for the speaking witness between discovering her truth and sharing her truth. The silent witness returns to her studio work.

Her inner witness:

> You must be
> looking
> for someone
> to hold you.
> You are all alone
> in this room.
> I want to hold
> you.
> Come to me.

◯ Imagining that her mover wants to be held could be an unconscious projection of her own feelings. Though awareness of projection begins in this discipline within the mover's practice, it becomes boldly apparent through the still looking of a witness presence. Here the silent witness is assuming that her own feelings of wanting physical contact are the mover's feelings. Rather than saying "This is my projection. . . . " I encourage her to ask herself: "How do I feel in the presence of someone who I believe wants to be held?" The silent witness discovers that she feels an overwhelming desire to hold this mover.

She keeps working.

Her inner witness:

> *You are a baby*
> *an abandoned baby.*
> *You are left here*
> *alone*
> *frantic*
> *that's why you crawl*
> *faster and faster.*
> *This is too hard*
> *sitting here*
> *and doing nothing.*
> *How can I tell you*
> *that I won't*
> *abandon you?*
> *I won't*
> *abandon you.*

◖ The silent witness realizes that she could be making an unconscious inter-pretation based on her own experience of infant trauma: the frantic baby wants to be held because she has been abandoned. Just as a beginning mover she was merged with her inner witness, now in the beginning of her witness practice she understands that she is merged with her mover. The ques-tion:"How do I feel in the presence of what I see as an abandoned baby?" brings the silent witness toward understanding her desire to scoop up, rescue, and soothe the abandoned baby within her own nervous system, her own psyche. If she were a speaking witness, unless the mover speaks of feeling abandoned, rather than saying "this is my story" or "this is what I think" she would contain her experience—a blessing, an opportunity for her to explore again her developing conscious relationship to her own infant trauma.

Silent witnesses discover more and more about themselves in the pres-ence of a mover.

A mover: I am crawling.

New silent witnesses:

> *I see you crawling.*
> *And you keep crawling*
> *you keep crawling.*

Their inner witnesses:

> *I see you crawling and:*

>> *I see an image of my baby sister crawling toward me. I see sparks of purple light darting around my solar plexus. My fin-gers pull in toward my thumbs. I am furious. . . . I always had to pick her up and care for her due to our mother's absence.*

or

*I hear my father shouting, a haunting
presence. My breath becomes shallow. It
is difficult for me to look directly at the
mover crawling. I turn my head a bit to
the right side and look sporadically out
of the corners of my eyes. The accident
when my younger brother crawled over
the edge of the precipice. . . . I can't look.*

or

*I cannot sit still. Suddenly my energy
drains out of me as if I am thawing.
Depressed, heavy, and dense, I have to
look at her . . . right here in front
of me. I must. I am about to see something I do not want to see.*

or

*I am incredibly sad. You are looking for
something that you have lost that is
of value. I think of my dearest mother
who is becoming so helpless and frightened as she loses her memory, too soon,
too soon. Tears come to my eyes.*

or

*I notice tension across my shoulders. I
feel weary, impatient. How can I witness
you, now, here in this studio, when I can
barely witness my daughter's recent
behavior, her confusion, her choices.*

◻ A witness's stories from the past, from the present, are abundant. Internally tracking these detailed and complex narratives evoked by the mover can be fruitful for the witness, potentially healing. But learning how to bring such dense and specific material into conscious relationship with the mover's experience is hard work. Discrepancies can be significant. While these essential distinctions between the experience of the mover and of the silent witness are being explored safely in the silent witness practice, the mover is protected from the not always loving and kind feelings of the witness, especially when the witness's own unresolved psychological complexes are stimulated.

For the mover, much of the witness' experience is uninteresting, too raw, too complicated, often experienced as an interruption of her own process. These stories are not useful unless they relate to the mover's consciousness of her experience and her readiness to speak it. The judgements, projections, and interpretations of these particular silent witnesses are unrelated to the mover's words spoken after moving: "I want more and more space in which to crawl. I want no one and nothing in my way as I explore my freedom, my capacity to move fast and close to the ground." Feeling and then understanding the difference between the mover's experience and her own, the silent witness becomes conscious of her separateness, her boundaries, bringing her toward a dialogic relationship with the mover.

As more conscious awareness develops within this silent witness, the urgency of her experience of being in the presence of a frantic abandoned baby wanting to be held dissipates. If she were a speaking witness she might be less likely to impose her own experiences onto the mover as she becomes clearer about them and brings them into conscious relationship to the mover's experience. Her practice of containment, which begins with sitting to the side of the space and not moving, extends into her study of the speaking time, learning what she might contain and what she might speak if she were a speaking witness. Conscious relationship requires two separate beings.

Her inner witness:

> *I cannot know*
> *your experience.*
> *I can only know*
> *my own*
> *in your presence*
> *because*
> *of your presence.*

The awareness of separateness for a silent witness can soon invite an awareness of a desire to change the mover's work. These unconscious or conscious wishes present new challenges to the longing to simply be present now.

Her inner witness:

> *I am tired*
> *of seeing you*
> *crawling*
> *around the floor*
> *in circles*
> *in circles.*
>
> *I want you to stop*
> *do something else*
> *find comfort*
> *be more creative*
> *make sounds*
> *be more careful.*
> *You could easily*
> *bump*
> *into the stone bowl.*

◘ Here, if the mover speaks of boredom or a search for comfort or a frustrating absence of her own creativity or a wish to make sounds or a fear of bumping into the stone bowl, the silent witness finds resonance with the mover. If she were a speaking witness, she might choose to share her feeling. When naming her feeling it is usually not helpful to speak of its source in her own personal history or to speak of her attached associations. All of this must be considered as the practice of discernment develops for the silent witness.

Her inner witness:

> *How can I be respectful*
> *of my own experience*
> *not betray it*
> *but learn how*
> *to contain it*
> *and*
> *within my longing*
> *to be genuinely present*
> *speak only*
> *what feels connected*
> *with you*
> *speak only*
> *what comes*
> *from loving kindness*
> *from a desire*
> *to experience compassion*
> *for you*
> *for me?*

◖ It is a blessing if what is finally spoken and how it is spoken actually results in the mover's feeling seen. Here it is the intention, the longing to see clearly, that carries a witness, with compassion for herself and her mover, into a commitment toward presence. Presence becomes a loving act.

With practice and time passing, the silent witness and I decide together when it seems appropriate for her to step into the practice of speaking witness. For the silent witness, readiness to become a speaking witness is not determined by an absence of judgment, projection, and interpretation regarding her response to her mover's work. It is determined by the silent witness's relationship to her developing consciousness of such phenomena. Within the specific path of a developing witness practice, each individual continues to commit to a movement practice.

The Speaking Witness

*Therefore the seeker will discriminate between the
things that tend to blur his vision and those that
clarify it; such essentially will be his "morality."*

SATPREM

◻ The moving practice begins to be experienced for both mover and witness as a ritual. Leaving the cushion, coming to the carpet's edge, making eye contact, gazing into the emptiness, closing the eyes, moving, opening the eyes, making eye contact, returning to the cushion—the clear and boundaried form marks what becomes ritual space. Such external clarity in boundary births new experiences of internal freedom to move as one must, discovering the unique and highly ordered rituals of the mover's inner world. Speaking and listening together after the movement creates a continuation of ritual, a similar sense of heightened awareness of all that longs to come into form, now into words.

From her studies as a silent witness, the new speaking witness comes toward the responsibility of not only committing toward being present while she witnesses her mover work but also commits toward being present afterward, in actually speaking with her mover. In her practice of discernment, choosing what and what not to say includes her awareness of the length of time they have been working together, the feeling of trust between them, and the actual content of the mover's work. Sometimes she is clear about her experience while witnessing the mover work but then after she hears the mover speak, she is reminded of other aspects of her witnessing experience of which she wasn't as aware. Sometimes she is not ready to speak sensitively about any aspect of her inner experience. Naming the physical movement invariably confirms the presence and generosity of her witness presence.

Just as it is for some new movers when they practice tracking, there can be a need for some speaking witnesses to name everything, every detail, to become engrossed in the order, to know the challenge of mapping. In continuing supervision the speaking witness can learn about balancing the speaking of fine detail with the knowledge that too much at certain times can become tedious for her mover and thus less related to the fullness of her attention during the time when they speak together.

Just as it is for some new movers, at first for some new speaking witnesses the intention to remember later what her mover is doing now and what her inner experiences are in response results in an awkwardness, as if she is being distracted from being present. However, as in the moving practice, remembering and then speaking her experience afterward opens the witness into relationship to what is happening inside her, inviting an extended consciousness of it. Once conscious, it can become integrated. Integration releases her from the effort to remember in the moments of witnessing.

There is much for a witness to remember. In describing many boundaries the witness is the primary guide for the unfolding of a session. She attends to the clarity, the safety, and the aesthetics of the physical space. She holds the clock, holding awareness of conscious time. She is responsible for her own psychological safety and for an awareness of her mover's. There can be times when a witness cannot feel a connection with her mover. In such moments she might notice an instinctual alertness or that she is working doubly hard to be present, for herself and for her mover. For a witness, an absence of feeling safe can be a signal concerning such a break in connection, and she must call the mover back to open her eyes and to return to her cushion. Talking together clarifies both the mover's and the witness's experience. Regardless of the mover's experience, if the witness does not feel safe she cannot offer an open presence.

The witness's relationship to suffering, her capacity to bring a compassionate enough presence to her own, marks the boundaries of the mover's work in a mysterious way. A mover can only work safely on an edge of discovery if she intuitively knows that her witness can hold even this. The witness's experience of suffering does not necessarily need to include the same content that the mover is exploring, but the witness's capacity to include a quality of darkness into which the mover might choose to descend must somehow be known to her mover. A witness can discover the difference between an empathic and a compassionate awareness in the presence of suffering. A compassionate witness accepts what is, remains nonattached, and expects nothing. Feeling completely connected to her mover, she can arrive into a space in which she herself is not suffering, even though she is in the presence of suffering. Learning to speak clearly from such a place is a blessing.

Under the midday sun two women appear at once, leaving their shoes and one large straw hat at the studio door. The three of us have been meeting for many months. The woman with the white shawl, arriving from her immersion in the silent witness practice, is the new speaking witness. The mover, because of previous practice in another discipline, has quickly developed an ability to track her physical movement and her inner experiences.

Because this skill is integrating itself, detailed tracking in this particular dyad is mostly useful for the mover when she is enveloped by new content that can create frustration, chaos, fear, or awe.

After we share a pot of tea the mover puts on her red woolen socks, which she always wears when she moves. She makes eye contact with each of us, walks to the carpet's edge, and first waiting, now steps in, brushing her hands down her back in a rhythmic motion. I am aware of the doves' song, of the afternoon light filling the stone bowl, of the one lilac blossom never cut, the petals dark and stiff.

I notice the bare feet of the woman with the white shawl as they are placed directly on the carpet, her legs open, her knees bent. I am suddenly struck by her alertness as she sits there on her cushion, her focus intently on her mover. She is here, intending to be present.

Her inner witness:

> *As I see your eyes*
> *I remember*
> *yesterday*
> *with my brother*
> *his eyes*
> *as he spoke*
> *of his wife.*
> *You wait and wait*
> *and now step in*
> *heel first.*
> *I remember*
> *his eyes.*
>
> *I see your hands*
> *brushing down*

your back
as you move
toward the center.
I remember
suddenly
that I must
make the long drive
back
to my brother
tomorrow.

I see you stopping
waiting again.
I must concentrate
be here
for you
with you.
Now seeing you
walking backward
helps me attend.
I always love
to walk backward.

Twenty minutes have passed and I see the mover open her eyes and make eye contact with her witness and with me. She returns to her cushion, silent for a few minutes before beginning to speak.

Waiting in the presence of the emptiness, with
one hand on my belly and one hand on my heart,
I step in. Brushing, rocking into the center, waiting
in stillness, a pull to the left and I'm swaying
around my planted feet. Another pull to the left,

still swaying, my mouth opens. I want to speak
and can't. Walking backward, I suddenly stop again.
I need eye contact and turning toward you, I open
my eyes, grateful for your presence.

The witness responds with a warm smile to the brief marking of one pool
after another. The mover continues.

I need to choose a few places to speak because
they are not so clear. After eye contact, I stand at
the carpet's edge a while because I need to look at
the emptiness as if I must look into it. My legs are
shaking just a little—you probably can't see this—
and my belly is tight. When I step in and brush
down the back of me with the back of my hands, I
am comforted by the sensation of my heels going
down first and by the sweet rhythm that appears.

As my head is pulled to the left and I circle
around myself I feel a rush of galloping sensations
coming up from my pelvis. The area around my
nose and eyes begins tingling. I have two experiences at once: I realize I have no tissue in my
pockets and I glimpse a small quilt, in soft hues,
floating in the space to the left of my head. I
know a sharp and unbearable pain in my heart. I
must walk backward. This walking into the space
behind me must be just like this. I must do this.

The speaking witness responds.

I see you walk to the carpet and wait, one hand on your
belly, one hand on your heart. I am not aware of your

legs shaking but I notice that my belly is tight. This sen-
sation relaxes as you rock into the space, heels first. The
rhythm stirs me, opens me to a sudden and vivid mem-
ory of my young son playing at an empty beach. I sit
up straighter as I see. . . .

I feel fear as I hear you speak of your little son.
Saying this now brings that shakiness I felt in the
beginning. I don't know. I need to move again.

As I light a candle to meet the changing of the mood my eyes meet the
mover's. The speaking witness, straightening the threads of her shawl with
her fingers, now makes eye contact with her and then takes a sip of tea.

Her inner witness:

Our eyes meet.
Perhaps I should
not have spoken
of my son.
I feel a wave of panic
not knowing
what I have done.
As you look
at me this time
I feel I am
being asked to help.
More panic.
How will I know
how?

I concentrate on
my own breathing

warding off
some fear.
This is a moment
of suspension
of trust
of complete not knowing.

The mover crawls to the edge of the carpet and sits down cross-legged, her hands in her lap, her head slightly tilted to the left. She sits there for ten minutes, opens her eyes and turns back to make eye contact with each of us. She now crawls back and sits in the same cross-legged position near us. After waiting and more waiting, she talks to her speaking witness.

> When we make eye contact in the beginning, I feel such longing, such helplessness. Soon I sit at the edge, waiting, feeling very teary. I feel my thumbs circling each other in my lap. I become very focused on the ungraspable nature of this particular gesture. I think maybe I'll do it forever.
>
> As I tilt my head to the left, my thumbs disappear. A dim nebulous field surrounds me. I see nothing, no shapes, no movement, nothing. For an instant I wonder if I exist. I don't know why but I feel fear. I am afraid nothing will happen. I'm afraid that something will happen. I am afraid of you both seeing me disintegrate, become out of control. I'm afraid of death. Inside I suddenly hear a voice that says "stop now." Both relieved and disappointed, I crawl back to you, feeling a trust in your presence.

Later in supervision the witness talks with me about her studio work in this session with this mover. We review her experiences as well as how she feels about what she has said. She speaks of feelings of guilt when her concern about her brother distracts her. She tells me of her worry in mentioning the memory of her own son and also her fear of not knowing if she could actually be helpful.

Now in the presence of her mover she does not speak about any of this and instead stays as close to the detail of her mover's words as she can. Here she responds by carefully choosing what to say from the authenticity of her own experience of these most recent ten minutes, using her mover's words as references, as places to mark her feelings of connection with her.

> When you crawl to the carpet's edge, I breathe way
> down into my pelvis. It is there that I notice a subtle but
> clear contraction in my pelvis. Now I see your hands in
> your lap, your thumbs circling and time opens. I am
> stunned by this tiny repetitive movement of your two
> thumbs. Yes, this gesture feels ungraspable for me too,
> especially within the enormity of this space and its
> emptiness that looms in front of us. As your head tilts I
> feel that there is enough time, enough space.

This dialogue continues to develop, to deepen, and it is time to end. I watch the two women walk down the brick path together, talking quietly, stopping briefly at the new sage plant. I am reminded to burn sage in the studio before the next mover arrives. I find dried leaves from the old and overgrown sage bush here just outside and beyond the deck. I place them into the little stone bowl made from a chip of marble from the carving of the large bowl in the corner. I bring fire to this vessel and slowly walk the circle of the room, beginning and ending here at my cushion. May this space become clear, newly opened, for whatever energy enters next.

Time passes. I see the mover walking up the path, turning to talk to the dove who likes to sit on the rim of the dog's water bowl. There is one red sock tucked into each of her hip pockets. The dove follows her to my studio deck and perches on the arm of the bench. As she comes inside and pulls the socks out of her pockets and onto her feet, the woman with the white shawl arrives and we begin. After thirty-five minutes of moving and witnessing, the mover first shapes the pools and now speaks in detail.

> Just standing in the presence of emptiness opens
> me, opens me to shaky legs, to a tightening belly,
> to fear. My mouth is suddenly dry, my heart is
> pounding. My mouth keeps opening and then
> closing. Pressure builds in my upper chest, wet
> sand pushing upward, but I have nothing to say. I
> feel helpless as I turn and walk backward into the
> space, toes first. There is no rocking, no sweet
> rhythm. I am walking backward. There is
> absolutely nothing else to do. I am walking back-
> ward, slowly.
>
> Here, just in this moment, I stop and turn around,
> simply arriving into the space behind me. Here I
> see so clearly my stillborn baby eight years ago. I
> am crying and whispering to him. No one must
> hear what I say but him. I tentatively pick him up,
> not taking my eyes off of him and just stand there,
> not knowing. My head turns to the left and a cry

erupts out of me that I've never heard before, one
sound.

Still holding my baby, I begin to walk more
deeply into that space behind me, that space
where I found him. Walking backward, he is still
mine. I keep him. Suspended, actually expanded, I
walk into another realm where everything is
transparent. The next thing I know I am at the
stone bowl, trembling as I bend down. I listen and
wait. Then I lay him in the vessel, cover him with
that little quilt in my mind, creating a ritual of
burial that never happened. I am shaken. I open
my eyes and see the emptiness in the bowl. I stand
and come back to you, seeing your wet eyes, seeing you with gratitude.

The mover and witness are silent together for a long time. The witness
touches her mover's hand as she speaks her experience of the end of the
mover's work.

I see your lips moving as you bend over and pick up a
bundle. Now I see the bundle is a baby. I know I am not
supposed to hear what you are saying. I wonder even if I
should not see, maybe look away because I am witnessing
an intimate moment. But I decide to look and I see you
clearly now speaking to this being, words I don't know or
need to know. Now I see you standing with an infant
and a wave of great sadness sweeps over me.

As you walk backward carrying this baby, I am also sus-
pended. I too am expanding as I gaze around the room,

my eyes marking the firmness of the walls, windows,
the floor and the stone bowl. Simultaneously I experience
all of these forms as transparent. A calmness comes over
me. Now you stop at the bowl and place your baby in it.
It is only in this moment that I know the baby is dead.
You cover him and my whole body relaxes. A necessary
ritual is happening. I am privileged to witness this
completion, to welcome you back, to be with you now.
I hear the doves calling.

The three of us talk quietly together for a while and it is time to say good-bye for now. As the women leave I realize that I need to go to the lilac tree here outside the window. I find the scissors and cut off the one blossom with the dark and stiff petals, dropping it to the earth, bringing order to my universe.

◻ Not only judgment, projection, and interpretation must be understood in the practice of witness consciousness. The realm of intuition, a potent place in human experience, must be respectfully addressed, especially for people for whom there is an innate and strong aptitude, as there is for this speaking witness. Until a witness is very practiced in tracking her experience of sensation, emotion, and thought, she is not usually prepared to recognize clear intuitive knowing as distinct from projective phenomena, disconnected memory forms, or ungrounded fragments of energetic phenomena. Extended commitment to the practice of clarifying experience based in psychological complexes usually precedes sharing intuitive experience with a mover. It does not seem helpful, respectful, or at times even safe for a witness to speak with her mover regarding "knowing" something about the mover of which the mover is not yet conscious. The conscious witness would choose to contain her intuitive experience, waiting until the mover is ready to address it. Here the witness feels she intuitively knows about the mover's experience.

The mover:

> I am crying and whispering to him. No one must
> hear what I say but him.

The witness:

> *I know I am not supposed to hear what you are saying.*
> *I wonder even if I should not see, maybe look away*
> *because I am witnessing an intimate moment.*

The witness is intuitively resonating with what the mover is doing and offers her witnessing because the mover speaks the moment and its quality first. In this situation the witness has an intuitive experience related to the mover's work but she herself is not experiencing the same thing. She is not *in* the intimate moment; in fact, she considers looking away from it. Here she is not in a unitive state with her mover.

When a witness is in a unitive state she consciously knows the experience of the mover because it is also her experience in the same moment. She is not merged with the mover because she is completely present, aware of what the mover is doing and of her own experience in response. The witness is not in a dialogic state with her mover because she knows a direct experience of wholeness, of nonduality. In a unitive state her boundaries are porous as she consciously experiences herself and her mover as the same, no longer two separate beings. This way of knowing, which includes intuition by definition, can be manifest in an experience of clear seeing, seeing without the density of emotion or thought. Here both the mover and the witness speak of being in a unitive state.

The mover:

> Suspended, actually expanded, I walk into another realm where everything is transparent.

The witness:

> *As you walk backward carrying this baby, I am also suspended. I too am expanding as I gaze around the room, my eyes marking the firmness of the walls, windows, the floor and the stone bowl. Simultaneously I experience all of these forms as transparent.*

Here both the mover and the witness have entered the same energetic field, the same world where the quality is specific, imbued with an experience of timeless and infinite space. Such experience of energetic phenomena can be distinguished from the experience of sensory and emotional energy related to personal history in which the person describes the opposite, the entrance into a specific place with no space around or outside of it. A unitive experience can consistently be distinguished from a dialogic experience because the individual, no longer identified with personal story, is no longer in relationship with time and space.

The Collective Body

Developing
Collective
Consciousness

All sorrows, without distinction, are ownerless;. . .
So why should the body of another not be taken as
my own?...Whoever wishes to quickly rescue
himself and another, should practice the supreme
mystery: the exchanging of self and other.

SANTIVEDA

Coming Toward the Circle

The colors of tulips and roses are not the same,
Yet in each we assent to the single Spring.

GHALIB

◐ Time passing, committed practice, hard work, and grace prepare us to widen the circle. From dyad to triad to quartet, the practice opens. Small groups, like a family, organically form as the longing to be part of something larger than oneself emerges. Moving from the foundation of dyadic practice does not mean that the need to be seen by another no longer exists. It means we are becoming more conscious of this longing, more able to be in dialogic relationship to it. The individual body and the collective body overlap, becoming interdependent as we learn to know ourselves as part of a whole.

Various configurations made up of different numbers of movers and witnesses both deepen the practice and directly prepare participants for entering the collective body work. When a witness works with more than one mover the external stimulation multiplies, demanding more awareness of the developing complexities of her own inner experience. She is tracking different and simultaneous movement series of others as well as her own experience, intending toward conscious relationship to each. It is natural for the witness to try to witness the movers equally. When it is time to speak together, the witness must guide the conversation so that there is time and space for each mover to speak her own work and her work in relationship with other movers and to receive witnessing.

While witnesses are learning to work with several movers at once, the number of moving witnesses grows, becoming a moving body. As members of a moving body, movers can experience joy in companionship and in belonging. They can also experience competition, jealousy, or fear of rejection. Because there is more than just one other mover, a mover with eyes closed might not literally recognize another mover whom she encounters, freeing her toward the possibility of experiencing a clearer slate for projections of internalized figures.

When a mover works with more than one witness she can experience the differences and similarities of what is offered and how it is articulated. In this format the mover can project her experiences of parents, siblings, or other primary figures in her life onto two or three witnesses. She can embody her projections safely in such a format, allowing the presence of more than one witness to affect her work.

While movers are learning to work with a growing number of witnesses, each witness is experiencing the witness circle widening. When the number of witnesses grows, witnesses can know uncomfortable feelings of competition or fear of being misunderstood as well as a deep relief in not having to feel solely responsible to see and articulate all that might be seen. Freedom begins to emerge as each feels accompanied by the presence of the others. They can learn of each other's experience of the same mover and how such experience is spoken.

As the family of movers and witnesses grows the inner witness within each person opens to include the outer presence of more personalities, requiring more awareness of inner layers of experiences intermingling and coexisting. Now the work in small groups both complicates and clarifies experiences of seeing and being seen, enriching the potential for consciously embodying that which is ready to be known.

Four women arrive under two umbrellas. The candle has been burning since I swept the floor in the early dawn. The doves' house is wrapped securely to keep the birds dry. The absence of their call is filled with the sounds of the rain on all of these windows. Sitting on the carpet, we drink tea as I explain the new guidelines of the work we will be doing this morning.

The beginnings of rounds are no longer marked by my voice, a symbol of the personal presence of a witness. Instead, I ring a small brass bowl once, the vessel and the sound becoming a symbol of something impersonal, connecting us to a larger whole. More freedom is available for witnesses now as they can consciously choose to stand up, exploring how a different visual plane might support or disturb their own concentration or that of other witnesses.

Today we begin a round of two witnesses and two movers. The witnesses are the woman with the white shawl and the woman with the red socks. The movers are the woman with the long gray hair and the woman with her black shawl tied today around her waist. All have extended practice as mover, moving witness, silent witness, and speaking witness within the dyadic and triadic formats.

I see the movers make eye contact with each other and now with their witnesses. I see the two witnesses, one in a chair, one on a cushion, looking at each other and then at me, acknowledging our mutual commitment to witness together. I ring the bell once as our attention turns toward the emptiness. After twenty minutes, I ring the bell three times to announce the end and we gather to speak and listen. Each mover acknowledges the shape of this round by naming her pools. Then, practicing the art of discernment, the mover with the black shawl speaks more specifically.

In transition between my second and third pool, I
am unfocused, crawling, not knowing where I am
going. Lowering my head slowly but with intention, my forehead touches down on the rim of the
bowl. This touch and I recognize myself, as if
yielding into my own presence. Settling on my
knees, I begin circling the edge of the bowl with
both hands as they tumble over each other.

Coming toward my own edge, my hands stop
moving. Enduring my own edge, I tentatively
place one hand, palm first, into the emptiness. I lift
it out quickly and go back to circling the edge of
the bowl. Again, I place one hand, palm first, into
the emptiness. This time I commit to this gesture
and I find the bowl not empty.

As the mover speaks here her voice becomes a whisper, her eyes close.

Feeling a need to hide while I move, I feel a need
to hide now as I begin to talk. My heart is pounding. Shards, broken shards . . . I am fingering shat-
tered pieces, uneven edges, a meager pile of dimly
colored forms. My shoulders come forward as I
lean my forearms on the edge of the bowl. I am
broken. All vestiges of a semblance of having it
together vanish. This is what I know and strangely
I know a relief in touching this truth. I am broken.

At this time in the practice we discover that we need to make it clear
when a person has finished speaking. We look for a natural gesture that
already seems to be emerging in the collective. Here the mover who has

just spoken places her hands, palms down, on the floor in front of her, allowing her torso to bow forward. She looks at each of us. Have we heard her?
As listeners we can choose to nonverbally acknowledge that we have heard
her words by making the same gesture and/or responding with eye contact.

The woman with the long gray hair now speaks the details of her experience more fully.

> Also somewhere in the middle of my work, I am
> on my toes and the top of my head is hot. This
> spot pulls my whole upper body down, arching
> me forward, until my hands touch the floor. I am
> aware of my breathing. Stretching my arms out
> farther away from my body, I see that my body is
> forming a specific shape, as if it knows how to
> create the correct container for an experience that
> is ready to be felt, seen, and heard. I hear myself
> make a sharp and high-pitched sound. My head
> begins to nod in a different, dragging rhythm.
> Here for the first time, I am accepting my father's
> death and the terrible way in which it happened. I
> instantly know that I cannot change my past but I
> can change my relationship to it. I see only emer-
> ald green. I am cleansed.

This mover lowers her hands onto the floor, acknowledging the end of her
time to speak. She remains in this position for a moment before coming
back up. Some respond by doing the same gesture with her, some quickly,
some more slowly. Now the woman with the red socks speaks as a witness,
first to the woman with the black shawl, responding to the place of work
which the mover has spoken.

As I see you exploring something in the bowl my own hands become unfamiliar, thick and large. I now find tracking your every gesture an essential grounding. I will try naming what I actually see because I feel such a long distance between my experience and words. I see your right hand in the bowl and your fingers and thumbs all coming together. As this hand lifts out of the bowl, I am ready to see what it holds. I am not afraid.

And now she speaks to the woman with the long gray hair, addressing her experience of the place that this mover has spoken.

Right as my hands are becoming so changed, I hear your high-pitched sound and feel it enter my feet and come coursing up my spine, into and out of my head, into the space above me. There it spins into a tunnel of brilliant colors. Your hair covers your face but I see your head slowly nodding, affirming, comforting me. Oddly, I begin to nod, as if I am comforting you.

We all place our hands on the floor in front of us, bending, taking in what has been offered, before the woman with the white shawl responds, first to the woman with the long gray hair and then to the woman with the black shawl, responding to the places marked by each mover.

I see you arched over, your hands flat on the floor. I, too, am aware of your breathing as I see the back of your torso slowly moving up and down. As you make the high-pitched sound, my eyes inside see the upper half of a sphere lift up and away from me, as though the top of my head is coming off. I am the one going up into the abundance of light and space. Simultaneously I see you

at the bowl fingering forms, holding shapes. I am also
the one in the lower half of the sphere, working at the
bowl, tending to what is just here in front of me. I am
whole, cleansed.

The dialogue continues into the morning as each woman unwraps another layer of her experience in the presence of the others. Near the end of our time together the two witnesses discuss their appreciation for each other, a shared relief in not being the only witness. One witness says in a certain moment in this morning's work she can see that the other witness is focused on that mover over there, which frees her to focus on this mover nearby. The witnesses also discuss a particular kind of intimacy that can occur when a mover is working very close to a witness. After the last woman speaks we all bow forward. Coming up and looking out, we see that the rain has stopped. We see rows of beads, raindrops shimmering, suspended along the length of the grasses just outside the big doors across the room. Green is glistening everywhere in wet light.

On this damp and bone-cold winter day the same four women arrive, ebullient in their greetings. Once settled and drinking hot tea, I introduce the new format: three people witnessing one mover. The woman with the long gray hair chooses to be the mover. The rest of us stay on the carpet as witnesses. I ring the bell once as the mover walks to the carpet's edge. After much eye contact she gathers her hair on top of her head and, laughing, marches in. Now letting her hair fall, she throws her arms straight up above her head. Thrusting her head back, her mouth opens wider as she continues to laugh. The laughing becomes louder, becomes new sounds, arrhythmic sounds, as she begins to toss her head out to her sides and now down toward the floor, her hair sounding as it hits.

Her inner witness:

> *All these witnesses*
> *all this freedom*
> *and I am a bit wild.*
> *I hurl my torso*
> *down and slap*
> *the floor.*
> *I swing my torso*
> *to my sides and around*
> *spinning and laughing.*

The witness with the red socks smiles and stands up.

Her inner witness:

> *I love this feeling in me*
> *when you swing*
> *throw yourself*
> *bang the floor.*
> *I love this freedom in me.*
> *I want this freedom in me.*
> *Gratitude. Gratitude.*
>
> *I want this.*
> *I want this.*
> *I crave this*
> *freedom in me.*

The woman with the white shawl sits closest to the wooden floor as she witnesses and now becomes focused on her own feet.

Her inner witness:

> *I can only listen.*
> *I can only listen.*
> *I feel the floor*
> *vibrating*
> *under my feet.*
> *I am too tired.*
> *I cannot look here.*
> *I am glad there are*
> *other witnesses.*

The third witness is crying as she smoothes her black shawl across her lap.

Her inner witness:

> *What is this?*
> *I feel overwhelmed*
> *with fear*
> *as I see this woman*
> *hurling herself*
> *around and slapping*
> *the floor.*
> *I cannot seem to stop*
> *my own tears.*
> *I am losing relationship*
> *I am merging*
> *with this mover.*

I ring the bell three times after twenty minutes of work. Witnessing the mover open her eyes, I see her looking out the window past the lilac tree into the hills far across the valley. She interlocks her hands behind her head and, dropping her head back into them, rests it there as tears fall. Soon she turns back toward us, looking into our eyes as she walks back to her cushion. I ask her to choose one place after marking the pools. She speaks now of the end of her work.

> At the end, I am still hurling and slapping. I am
> surprised by a huge figure in front of me. I feel his
> feet under my hands as I slap the floor. I follow
> his outline up and know it is my son. He is solid
> and warm, receptive and strong, forgiving. Here in
> his presence, I know he forgives me. Can I forgive
> myself?

Not looking at anyone, she lowers her eyes and her torso toward the floor. Others make the same gesture and then we are silent for awhile. Now the witnesses practice discernment as they move from the silent voices of their inner witnesses to speaking as outer witnesses, responding to the place in the work which the mover has chosen. One woman speaks of witnessing the mover's hands following the outline of a human form in front of her and her own experience of someone else arriving in the room. Another witness speaks about not being able to look and then looking. She feels like she is in a sacred hut, looking out. She sees a ritual as an old woman stands before a young woman and exchanges something with her. She doesn't know what is being exchanged but she knows it is of value. The third witness says she is choosing not to speak at this time.

Not speaking is one of the benefits of having more than one witness. Different witnesses, with at times remarkably different experiences of the same mover, can share the responsibility. This woman's silence protects her and her mover from her own speaking prematurely. Later, in supervision, there is time for the woman with the black shawl to safely explore her experience of losing her boundaries, of not being able to contain her emotions while witnessing. Her inner witness strengthens as she becomes conscious of her own material in relationship to her mover's work, enabling her to both contain and honor her feelings.

I remember seeing the moon rise into the twilight yesterday evening. Now this morning, still full but so much more quiet in its light, it floats above the hillside. Under one moon, one witness, the woman with the black shawl, holds the space for three movers. She rings the bell once as we all acknowledge each other with our eyes. Twenty minutes pass and she rings the bell three times.

In preparation for speaking together I ask people, when referring to a specific mover, to say "a mover" or "another mover" rather than naming the person or even looking at her. This guideline protects the mover by reminding the one who is speaking of the distinction between a mover's personality and her actual movement experience. It also protects the mover's timing. If she is not named the anonymity reduces feelings of obligation to respond. Also, if a witness says: "When I hear a mover crying, I discover my own sadness," there might be two movers crying and both can receive this witnessing in their own unique ways because neither has been named.

Now we sit in a circle on the floor waiting for each mover to begin speaking. Pools are named. The woman with the white shawl speaks now, beginning with her eyes closed.

> I walk in and immediately realize that I do not have to stand up! I am sucked down and around my own center, propelled into the floor, stretching long and onto my belly. I can hear another mover's chanting, feel her presence, but I am pressing my body into the floor, especially my forehead and my hands near my head. I am filling with grief as my heart opens. Here I am coming nearer to myself. I have been too far away from myself. This clear chamber without walls is always here, but I remember that I forget to reside within it. I must stay here now. I am clear when I am alone and not so clear when I am in relationship. I need to be alone. When I stand up at the end, I look down and see an imprint of my body on the floor. I don't want any witnessing.

The mover with the long gray hair speaks next.

> I also am coming home. But first I am pulling little hard knots of pain out of my chest. The more I pull, the larger they become—larger, harder, uglier. I throw them into the room, I pound them into the floor, stomping, heels down, slashing, arms

cutting, here in front of me, there to the side of
me, shouting. I am shouting, biting, roaring. I am
fury. I am mad. What a relief to fulfill this impulse.

Now the last mover speaks as she pulls her arms around her bent legs, dropping her chin into the crevice formed by the meeting of her knees. Her
hands caress her feet, which are covered in her red wool socks.

> I sit at the stone bowl, feeling it especially along
> the inside of my thighs as I wrap my legs around
> it. I hold it. It holds me. I listen to another mover
> shouting. At the same time I am becoming more
> and more silent, sipping the emptiness inside the
> stone bowl. My hair dips into the void, at first
> with a delicacy. Dipping, blissfully dipping, I begin
> to chant. I chant into it, it chants me back.
> Humility sweeps into me as a membrane silently
> tears and I see lights filling what is becoming a
> vessel of incomprehensible proportions, of incom-
> prehensible beauty. In awe, I begin weeping and
> cannot stop. Perhaps I too am coming home.

The mover with the long gray hair continues.

> Finally, with nothing left to discard, I become still,
> emptied. It is here that I come home. I think I am
> on my knees. My hands arrive into a great silence
> in front of my chest. My wrists are together, my
> fingers cupping up and around an empty space. I
> decide to pull them apart but they snap back
> together. Again and again, they snap back together.
> It is as though this gesture, invisibly present in the

moving space, insists on embodiment. I wonder if
it is up to me to discover and enter it so that the
gesture itself can remember embodiment, remember its source.

The only witness listens to what each mover says, bending her torso down
toward the floor with each one as movers complete their speaking. She
gives in-depth witnessing to only two of the movers, respecting the third
mover's request.

▢ Movers often discover places of awe or beauty in what surrounds them
just before closing their eyes or while moving in the light or stroking the
smooth wooden floor. Sometimes movers, like the woman coming into a
unitive state with the light, experience the beauty and the awe as inseparable. The moment of eyes opening after immersion in an inner world of
movement experience can also bring a mover into a startling awareness of
the beauty of things as they are all around her.

Beauty and awe appear and disappear as immediate gifts in this work,
as blessings. The insistence, the recurrence of movement patterns, often
appear and disappear not only as challenges but as blessings as well. As time
passes some movement patterns and themes become resolved and disappear.
Others continue to reappear in surprising moments. And still others continue with a consistent and tenacious demand for more attention. It is the
development of the inner witness in relationship to such work that
becomes a guiding force in determining an individual's readiness for entering a larger group, not an absence of movement patterns or psychological
complexes.

The longing to be seen by another and to see another open toward a
longing to participate within a whole, to discover one's relationship to many
without losing an authentic or truthful awareness of oneself, without betray-

ing oneself. With stronger and clearer inner witnesses people prepare to bring experience of the ground form into a circle of movers and witnesses.

Readiness for a larger group reflects a growing awareness of a desire to belong. Exploration of such a longing opens individuals toward questions of the relationship between the self and the collective. The embodiment of collective consciousness can only become manifest because of the embodiment of personal consciousness. If we abandon such essential ground by sacrificing or manipulating the personal voice in order to feel as though we belong, we do not truly belong, we are not truly whole. And if we ignore the opportunity for consciously embodied membership we heighten our sense of alienation, isolation, and despair, all of which insidiously and profoundly disable us as individuals.

One Circle

*Before the creation of the world, Ein Sof withdrew
itself into its essence, from itself to itself within
itself. It left an empty space within its essence,
in which it could emanate and create.*

KABBALAH

Walking into the hills early this morning I find the pussy willows just beginning to bud. Gathering a huge bouquet of them I bring this sign of new spring into the studio, placing them in a tall vase on the window seat inside the door. Six people arrive just on time, one woman taking off her jewelry and hanging her earrings on one of the branches. There are four women: the one with the white shawl, the one with red socks, the one with the black shawl, and the one with long gray hair. Two men are also in this group, one tall, the other one bearded, both arriving with extensive practice in the preceding formats. All of these people have practiced for many years in this studio and some have been practicing here with each other for a long time. A labyrinth of memories arrive with each one of us as we embark on a new way.

Now we begin.

Sitting together in this circle on the wooden floor our bodies form the edges of an emptiness before us, reflecting our potential experience of emptiness within. Opening toward the mysteries of filling and emptying this circle we are opening toward an exploration of the relationships between movers and witnesses, among witnesses who are witnessing at the same time and among those who are moving at the same time.

In this new circle the practice of concentration continues to ground and enliven the developing relationship between the moving self and the inner witness. We begin by bringing the dyads into the collective body. Three movers will now be participating in a moving body, each one continuing to have the security of his own witness. Three witnesses will be participating in a witness circle, each one focusing just on one mover. In this way, everyone, with some preparatory practice in quartets, can become familiar with the energy of many movers and many witnesses practicing in the same circle.

When witnesses remain in one place they are strengthening the form of the circle itself. Try not to move around, even if it seems that you might see your mover more easily from a different perspective. Practice receiving the perspective that is offered, even when your view of your mover is blocked by another mover. When movers return they will know to find their witness exactly where they were when their eyes first closed and movement began.

When we begin, stretch your arms wide to your side, actually making the shape of the circle more vivid, both visually and energetically. As you do this try to make eye contact with each person. I will ring the bell as we bring our attention to the emptiness. When you are ready, every other person will become a mover, starting here with you on my right. The person to the right of each mover will be that mover's designated witness. Before movers close your eyes, make eye contact with your witness and with the other movers. Witnesses, after connecting with your mover, make eye contact with the other witnesses, acknowledging your shared commitment.

I ring the bell once and we begin by bringing our attention to the emptiness. As the teacher, knowing that each mover has a designated witness, my gaze lingers on the face of each person here. I wonder about the inevitability of our paths in relationship to our will, to our intention toward conscious choice.

My inner witness:

> *I am bathed*
> *in gratitude.*
> *I can see*
> *the focus of each*
> *witness*
> *on a mover.*
> *Every mover*
> *has a witness.*
> *Every*
> *mover has*
> *a witness.*
>
> *I see the bearded man*
> *seated*
> *his legs crossed*
> *witnessing near*
> *the stone bowl.*
> *Light streams*
> *into that empty vessel*
> *near him*
> *changing the color*

of his hair.
May light stream
into this empty
vessel
this circle
carved by the shapes
of our bodies
here
in this moment
in this time
in this space.

May we each see
ourselves
and each other
a little more
clearly.

Forty minutes have passed. Signaling the end, I ring the bell three times. Each mover comes out of the circle, attending to the transition from inner toward outer awareness, making eye contact with the other movers and with her or his own witness. After making eye contact with their movers, witnesses make eye contact with each other and we again witness the emptiness. Now each dyad speaks together while the whole group listens. In guiding the dialogues I ask the mover to first silently name sequential pools of movement and then to choose one place to speak in more detail. I ask the witness to respond, staying as close to the mover's experience as possible.

Now the circle begins again: people reach out to ground and embody the circle, make eye contact, and witness the emptiness. Those who were movers become witnesses and witnesses become movers. As movers come out, making eye contact with their witnesses, we all again witness the emptiness, completing the round of work. People speak together in dyads as the group listens. The strength of the inner witness is especially called upon here when, for the first time within one session, movers and witnesses switch roles with their partners, changing perspective from seeing to being seen, from being seen to seeing. It is inevitable that the witness is affected by the mover and the mover by the witness, so the next round always begins with visible and invisible hues of the last round. Because of this, some receive a first glimpse of a knowing that mover and witness consciousness are potentially the same.

◧ In this first circle new ways of experiencing the self appear. In the mover's practice the urgency to be seen can begin to shift toward a desire to participate. Movers want to know how their experience relates to what other movers are doing, asking: "How do I fit in?" One can learn that the fullness of personal experience can coexist with other movers and witnesses discovering their own truth. The circle becomes a fertile place, what can be experienced as a necessary place, for every mover. There must be a place for the one who begins and ends in one position, never moving. There must be a place for the one who fills the space with constant movement and sound, for the one who goes from mover to mover searching for contact and for the one who needs to be near a witness. There must be a place for the one who chooses not to speak, for the one who speaks with an unclear or frustrated voice, for the one who can see himself clearly, and for the one who cannot.

Witnesses become engaged with new questions. "How do I work with a desire to protect my mover from other more active or noisy movers? How can I stay present for certain movements that repel, frighten, sadden, or bore me? How do I remain unattached to certain movements that I experience as exquisitely beautiful or ones that stir my soul? When I lose a feeling of connectedness with my mover, how do I prevent myself from shifting from a practice toward presence into an experience of voyeurism? How do I bring awareness to all of this and simultaneously stay connected with other witnesses?"

A hummingbird, gorgeously green and suspended among the rosemary flowers, appears just as the six people come along the path. We marvel at her capacity to drink while suspended in midair. Once inside, we share a pot of tea and begin the work. I speak about a new format emerging from an individual readiness to move and witness without designated dyads. We begin with everyone sitting in the witness circle. As the teacher, I will remain a constant witness.

This new circle feels long and open, spacious in welcoming each of you to follow your inner timing, directly choosing from moment to moment to become a mover or to become a witness. The voice of the witness/teacher, the bell ringing, the format itself no longer determine when it is time to be a mover or to be a witness. In this long circle, for what can be an extended period of time, people are constantly changing roles, following a call to move or a call to witness.

Spontaneously changing roles invites a wakefulness, a possibility of moving at any second, requiring attention toward a continuous flow between movement and stillness. You can move for five minutes, witness for twenty, move for one minute, witness for ten, move in and out and in and out within seconds, embodying the question of right timing, or you can move the whole time. To ensure a strong and safe enough witness circle for such a dynamic moving body, a new guideline is introduced for witnesses becoming movers. Including the teacher, there must always be a certain number of witnesses, the number decided upon by the collective before beginning the round. A mover's practice of discernment in consciously choosing how long to move is strengthened by this guideline, reminding him that at any time a witness might be waiting to become a mover. As the teacher, I will be a constant witness.

One reason a witness chooses to move can be because of his experiences directly related to witnessing a specific mover or movers. If there are enough outer witnesses he can choose to close his eyes and take these experiences immediately into his moving practice, expressing them rather than containing them within a witness perspective.

If you are witnessing and a mover is working behind you, even turning to look can disturb the concentration of the witness circle. Witnesses on the other side of the circle can see behind you and you can see what is happening behind them. We need the other half to see the whole. When the witness circle continues to be a consistently embodied shape, movers are free to work not only inside the circle but on the edge between two witnesses or outside the circle. Though every witness tries to welcome each mover with eye contact whenever he returns to his cushion, now movers give themselves permission to choose not to look at a witness if they are feeling too vulnerable or not ready.

With no designated witness for each mover and with many moving at the same time, the presence of the inner witness must strengthen to include the possibility that a person might not be seen in the way that he desires. It is an intention of witnesses to be present for all that arises and yet, because witnesses are human, it does not always happen. But movers, because they are human, desire that their witnesses offer full presence and unconditional love. Everyone now is called upon to bring a spirit of equanimity toward all others in the group, trusting enough the intention of the inner witness in each person and in oneself.

As the format changes, new questions appear. No longer depend-ent on an external signal to determine when you move or witness, what is your way of choosing to move? When you become a mover, how do you enter, where do you go in relationship to the circle, and how do you return to your place? What is your experience of so many others in the moving body with you—their sounds, their touch, their changing presence? What is it like to imagine or to be the only mover in a circle of witnesses? What is it like to imagine not being witnessed because of the work of another mover or movers which might be calling the attention of the witnesses?

As a witness do you respond to several movers at the same time or do you find yourself focusing on just one mover, or do you con-sciously choose to stay engaged with each one simultaneously? How do you feel in relationship to movers who are near you and to those who are farther away, to those who are quiet and to those who are sounding, to those inside and outside the circle? Here, you can deepen your exploration of choosing not to move, remaining a witness, containing your inner experience.

As the moving and witnessing time becomes longer and therefore more complex, a time of silent transition becomes natural before speaking together. For some, walking or resting is appropriate. For others, writing, drawing, or working with clay can clarify experi-ence. After the transition I will invite only the movers to speak from the voices of their inner witnesses. Outer witnesses are being asked to be silent once again, an opportunity to which we often return in the evolution of this practice. Hearing only movers' experiences helps witnesses in their developing practice of discernment, choos-ing what and what not to speak within this newer context of col-lective body work.

We now work for fifty minutes, followed by a transition in silence, bringing a different mood to the studio. Each person is alone, focused and yet next to another who is also alone and focused. I find myself walking the circle, counterclockwise, around and around, sometimes stopping to speak quietly with a participant about his work. As we gather in a circle, preparing to speak and listen together, I offer a few more guidelines.

Practice in tracking your own chronology as a mover or of another's movement as a witness prepares you for tracking your experience of the chronology of the group. When you speak, speak with an inner awareness of when your movement might have appeared not only in the sequence of your own work but within the sequence of the group's work. We will start with what feels like the beginning, adding moments from different movers as they seem sequentially related. At times in this process, those who speak are responding to content instead of sequential order. If one mover says: "I must stay with this loneliness," another might speak in response with a similar experience: "I also am aware of being lonely." Threading through both chronology and content clarifies the experience of becoming a conscious member of a collective body.

Begin your talking by saying "I am the one who," reminding us all, every time one person brings his experience into the circle, that we each are a part of a whole whether we experience it that way or not. If you do not wish to speak, say: "I am the one who is not ready to speak" or "I am the one who wishes not to speak." Listening to others is a significant contribution, a way for each of us that is always available for study and practice.

If you do not speak as a mover you will not receive verbal witnessing. The silence of your witnesses is an honoring of your silence.

Without your words as guidance in relationship to their own experiences, the risk of imposing their words is greater, possibly complicating or disturbing your experience before yours is formed enough.

Movers choose what to speak and choose what not to speak from the fullness of their experiences. After they speak, they make the brief gesture of bending toward the floor. Some who listen choose to respond with the same gesture, others do not.

The woman in the red socks speaks first.

> I am the one who steps into the circle, my heart
> racing. While standing, I find myself taking off my
> socks. Bending now in front of each person, as my
> hands shake, I realize I am sweeping the space in
> front of them with my precious socks. I need to
> do this.

The woman with the long gray hair speaks next.

> After my space has been cleared, I am the one
> who rolls into the emptiness as though I am
> descending into my own vastness. I lie here and
> lie here on my back, becoming very still, receiv-
> ing. My hair covers my face, bringing a delicious
> darkness, a deep peace.

The woman in the red socks speaks again.

> After preparing the space, I am the one who is
> lost, finds no movement that feels right. Lying on
> my side, I am eroding, becoming lifeless. I cannot

initiate anything. I feel a foot suddenly at my head.
Bringing my hand to this foot, now clinging to it,
I hear the sound of the heel being pulled away.
I let go feeling the agony of disconnecting,
of separateness, of not belonging.

After a long silence, the bearded man speaks.

> I am the one who enters the circle realizing there
> are only two of us men. I am also lying on my
> side, but in a cave, the same cave that I discovered
> as a mover years ago, the cave that held the dark-
> ness and density of my childhood. Now I arrive in
> this cave simply for shelter. I see images of peo-
> ple's faces, one after the other, as I "look" through
> the door. I am here, trusting, feeling connected,
> not alone.

Now the tall man speaks.

> Yes, as the other man I am the one who feels my
> power in this small room. Long and strong, I feel
> like an eagle. I have the immense sky, the immense
> view. I am alone in the sky.

Closing her eyes, the woman with the long gray hair speaks again.

> Out of the stillness my hands begin to stroke my
> body, touching my arms, breasts, belly and thighs,
> my feet and my face. My fingers comb through
> my hair, now touching my mouth. I know a lus-
> cious pleasure as I move into these new, sensual
> experiences. It has taken so long, too long to

know this kind of loving, loving being a woman, loving being in this body.

The tall man speaks again.

> I love being an eagle, feeling the strength of my
> wings, flying with my own great pleasure. I am
> free, euphoric, and finally strong again. I can feel
> my strength coming back, in my arms, my wings!
> And in my thighs and calves. Even my hands are
> strong again . . . and facile.

With his eyes closed, the tall man is slowly opening and closing his hands in front of his chest as he speaks. In this moment, he becomes teary.

> Yes, I am becoming strong again, finally becoming
> strong after my long illness. May I always be in a
> state of perpetual gratitude.

After some silence, the woman with the white shawl speaks next.

> With caution, I am the one who crawls into the
> circle with so much longing, weeping. I stay down
> on the floor close to a seated witness, rocking over
> my knees. I am shocked to realize that my longing
> is a prayer, my rocking is a prayer. Praying, and a
> bit self-conscious, I open to my own quiet mur-
> murs, tender and new.

Now the woman with the black shawl speaks.

> Becoming a moving witness, I find the woman
> who is weeping. Finding her, I find my own grief,

here just behind my face. Afraid of imposing, I touch her back, now her shoulders with both hands. Feeling welcomed, I receive her warmth, her breath, her closeness to me and I wrap my arms around her, making a safe enclosure for our tears. My feelings of aloneness fade as I hold her and allow her to hold me.

The woman with the white shawl speaks once more.

Being held, holding, rocking, and praying, I begin to sing a wordless song. I sing in celebration, not for the God in the universe but for the God in me. Singing, I suddenly and vividly know that this God is the same as the one in the universe.

Now the bearded man speaks.

I am the one who needs your song, really hears your song, leaves my cave and crawls out toward the center because of your song. My hand lands on an outstretched arm that is moving up and down. Now standing at the back of this great bird creature, my arms along the back of his arms, I am inspired. I want to soar, to risk letting go. I don't know how. I've never known how. My shoulders collapse forward as I recognize a familiar, crushing sensation in my chest. I withdraw and become a witness.

The tall man speaks.

I am the one who, when landing back here in this group from my eagle flight, feels disoriented and alone. I am sad when the mover behind me leaves just when I return.

The woman with the long gray hair speaks again.

> Basking in, breathing in, drinking in this pleasure, this "I love being in my woman's body" pleasure, I prepare to come out to witness because I begin to worry that I have been a mover too long. As I open my eyes I see two movers holding each other. I have been surrendering to the experience of my own touch. I am the one who feels a profound connection between them and me. It's as if loving myself does not separate me from others. I am not alone.

The woman in the red socks speaks now.

> Suddenly waking to the sounds in the room, I realize that I am the one who has been sleeping. Now I remember sleep coming from the tip of my tailbone, up my spine, over the top of my head, and into my center. Now the numbness is gone. I am refreshed.

◖ After we formally end the round of work, the woman with the black shawl wants to speak of her experience as a silent witness for most of the round. She says she is amazed at the fullness of what happens, at her relief and gratitude to again feel no responsibility for speaking to movers. She describes how deeply connected she feels with each mover. She tells us that this time she realizes that she doesn't need to speak her experience. "My desire for presence is enough."

Sometimes a mover actually falls asleep. Perhaps this long circle is the only safe place to sleep. Or maybe the mover needs to test the witnesses' commitment. Or it is possible that sleep is an appropriate response to a discovery of a frightening or disturbing experience. When a witness sees a mover sleeping, he might feel peaceful and relieved or angry and manipulated. Or he might be aware and respectful of the possibility of an invisible or visible catalyst that sends the mover to sleep. He might enjoy the possibility that someone is holding the place of the dreamer or he might be reminded that sometimes someone holds the place of the one who is not consciously experiencing himself as part of the collective body.

Though community building richly occurs in the moving and witnessing practice, it is not the primary intention of collective body work. The intention is toward participation in a consciously embodied collective. Participants choose to enter the circle for an infinite number of reasons or, at times, for no reason at all. People enter when they are tired or at peace, scared or depressed, hungry for pure movement or unable to sit still any longer. They enter because of a glance from another person here in the studio, a shift in the light, an insect landing near a foot, or the intense purple of the princess flowers, vivid beyond the window seat.

Here, in this studio on this day, as in life anywhere on any day, experiences happen simultaneously that are vastly different from each other. One is alone, one is not alone. One feels a sense of belonging and another does not. Longing, belonging, soaring, withdrawing, sleeping and waking, individuals take turns descending into different aspects of being human in the presence of each other. Consciously embodying one's truth in the presence of others can create an experience of wholeness, belonging, and completion as well as an experience of incompletion, frustration, and alienation. "I am because you are" seems true regardless of our experience of suffering or freedom from suffering.

Time passes, commitment deepens. The inner witness becomes increasingly stronger and more accepting of oneself and therefore of others. Language that naturally surfaces from conscious embodiment names this love. Presence becomes this love.

Autumn burns. The last person to arrive hops up onto the small deck after throwing one more ball for the dogs. This group continues to meet, now once a week for three-hour sessions. People come to the circle as they are, with stiffness or exhaustion, joy or fear or whatever they are experiencing in response to the demands and gifts of their current lives. We begin as we are rather than dispersing such fullness through movement warm-ups or verbal check-ins. Such preparation can disturb the intention for movers and witnesses to open toward what arises, toward no agenda, toward an absence of a preconceived theme or stated problem. At times both movers and witnesses are surprised to discover experiences that feel unrelated to what was assumed would emerge. I often feel that there are not just seven people here, but infinite numbers of others mysteriously manifesting a fragment, a remnant, a lightness or a darkness through the embodiment of those present.

The bell rings. We reach toward each other, make eye contact, witness the emptiness, move and witness for an hour, make eye contact, and witness the emptiness once again. Now the guidelines shift once more and the voices of the outer witnesses are included in the chronological and contextual weaving of the individual experiences being spoken. Here witnesses speak their experience of a mover's work if the mover has spoken it and also of their experience of witnessing in general or in becoming a mover, changing roles. The woman in the red socks speaks first, followed by a witness speaking.

> I am the one who walks the inner edge of the circle, my hands covering my empty womb.

>> *I am the one who sees a woman walking just in front of each witness in the circle. I want to walk with her but choose to witness instead. Suddenly I realize that this is exactly what I do with my therapy clients, contain so much of my experience. Here I have a choice. I am here.*

Other movers speak, each followed by a witness.

> I am the one who blesses my shawl in front of the stone bowl. With slightly opened eyes, I place it on the shoulders of the one who is walking around the inside edge of the circle.

>> *I am the one who sees a shawl being held over the stone bowl as if it is being blessed. I am uncomfortable with this gesture but try to be respectful of the mover doing what she needs to do.*

> I am the one who gladly receives a shawl. As my head falls forward, I remember my red socks on

my feet. I see fire. I see blood everywhere. I go to the windows, my hands stretched high. I smear the blood down the glass, onto the floor, all over the floor. Too much blood. Blood is everywhere on this earth. A particular pain surges up from my pelvis to my heart. I move into the center.

> *I am the one who is still choosing to witness, still choosing to contain. I see a mover wiping her hands down the glass. I imagine a viscous substance all over this room. Now I see her step into the center, her shawl covered in darkness.*

I am the one who finds a mover in the center of the circle and respectfully takes the shawl from her. I wonder: Is this the one I didn't like seeing blessed at the bowl? I wear the cloth to hide my identity, to find myself. Beneath its darkness, I wander unselfconsciously through a community.

> *I am the one who sees a tall man entering the circle, slowly lifting a black shawl from a mover's shoulders and then covering his face with it. I would like to be under that darkness right now.*

Here another witness speaks.

> *I am the one who sees a man covered in a black shawl and I am afraid.*

Now a mover speaks followed by two different witnesses.

Wearing the shawl, I am the one who is freed from the shame, from the shame of having a face, from the obligation to have a face. My face makes many faces, moving of their own accord, authentically and spontaneously, unseen by the witnesses. Am I too ugly, too despicable to be seen, or does every creative spirit require a mask to reveal himself?

Sitting as a witness, I am the one who feels nothing, knows nothing, finds no meaning in anything. We're simply men and women sitting and moving around in this room. I stand up.

I am the one who is still choosing to witness, still choosing to contain. I see a witness suddenly stand up.

A man now shifts from being a witness to becoming a mover.

Standing up, I now know that witnessing is not working. . . .

Standing up, I am the one who suddenly moves in running. Running, now dancing, my feet are drumming. It's the rhythm, my body remembers this rhythm. I am delighted, transported. Quicker, quicker, faster, faster, I don't want to stop.

A woman also shifts from witness to mover.

I am the one who sees one man dancing
near another man whose face is covered with
a cloth. That one looks like death to me. I
don't want death here. . . .

I enter the circle, wrestle the cloth off of him with
determination, only to discover that I am holding
him, holding life in my arms. Shaking, I go to the
floor, a feverish intensity swelling through layers
of moving forms and colors. Under these ethereal
slices of reality I see an exquisitely luminous ring
floating. Undulating vibrations pulse through the
ring and on up and through me, my skin becoming
permeable. There is much heat and pulsing in my
hips, spread legs, and through my spine and throat.
Opening my eyes to help me ground, I see two
people, one on each side, holding the shawl above
me. I see a *chuppah,* a canopy of sacred colors, as I
call out into the space. I hear drumming.

Another mover speaks.

I must keep dancing this intoxicating rhythm. I
am the one who becomes part of some ritual or
ceremony, drumming this dance with my feet,
drumming, drumming. My legs, my legs. Harder,
faster, my legs, my breath. I dance. I feel some fear
of erotic energy building. I risk really feeling it,
dancing it until the dance is done. I am here. The
fear is gone. I finally soar. I soar. I am free.

I am the one who sees the man
dancing. I have been waiting for this.

I see the shawl lifted up high. I see a
ceremony, an offering. I feel hope.

The following movers speak, some as moving witnesses.

> My clients are not here! I am the one who, with
> my heart pounding and an unfamiliar sense of
> fear, finally jumps in. Once in, with my eyes open,
> I turn to each witness and make eye contact,
> needing an extra hit of their presence. Closing my
> eyes, I stand, not knowing what I must do—as if I
> should always be doing something.

> Exposed, no longer protected by the dark cloth, I
> am the one who needs another man. I blindly go
> from mover to witness, touching faces, looking for
> him. I pause, stroking the softness of a woman's
> face, soaking in her feminine presence.

> I am the one who feels a man's hand lightly
> stroking my face. Instantly I am in the presence of
> my gentle father, my beloved father. My first
> reunion with him since he died too long ago
> when I was too young. I know this moment as
> grace. Gratitude, gratitude.

> Very sad to leave, I am the one who continues on
> my journey, still looking for the other man. I find
> his bearded face and abandon myself with him, my
> friend, my fellow man. I surrender to sheer physi-

cality, competing with all of my energy. I am here.
I am met. I am met! I am so grateful. I am met.

I am the one who throws my arms around his
belly. I ride him in fury and passion. Arms
stretched, fingers locked, my belly toward the sun,
we ride down, burrowing into the earth. Now we
release each other back to the circle. Carrying the
circle within me as we moved, now I need to see
the witness circle around us as we, the last movers,
come out.

◖ The circle is now becoming the external form of the practice. Just as in
the dyadic work the mover internalizes the outer witness, now movers and
witnesses internalize the circle as they fill and empty it. As the circle grows
inside each person, the mystery of the emptiness witnessed in the beginning and end of each round of work comes into deeper relationship with
that which is stirring within and emanating from each person.

Some witnesses, as their work develops, choose to return to the
beginning practice of saying only what they see. We begin the discipline
with tracking just physical movement and slowly become fully engaged
with the richness of inner experience. As the complex experiences of sensation, emotion, and thought are consciously embodied and therefore
integrated, they begin to take up less space in the psyche. When the witness in this round says *"I see a witness suddenly stand up,"* she is discovering
that such marking is enough, truthful because she is indeed experiencing
fewer sensations and emotions. Her personality becomes less responsive
and her experience of presence becomes more acute.

Sometimes a mover will receive witnessing from more than one witness and sometimes he will not receive any witnessing. In the absence of

response it can be tempting to ask for witnessing. A mover might have in fact been seen, but asking places a demand on witnesses who might not be ready to offer witnessing for any number of reasons, even if those reasons are not yet conscious. As the witness/teacher, it is my practice to ask the mover to endure, explore, trust what he experienced while moving and what he is now experiencing without witnessing. The work until now has encouraged constant protection of the mover in support of the developing inner witness. This continues, and at the same time the needs of the witness in the collective body work become more visible.

In the speaking time some speak, some do not. Though chronology and context usually guide the braiding of the larger narrative, sometimes an individual chooses to respond to another's speaking by addressing how he feels now in this moment of listening. He might respond with joy, confusion, or humor. As people practice speaking in a collective, specific words and phrases, like "I am here," once offered and genuinely received, begin to belong to the collective, shaping and refining a common language. A shared vocabulary reflects an experience of belonging and, at the same time, the direct, known experience of belonging becomes reflected in a language created in the presence of others. Each circle discovers a distinct but subtle way of speaking together. And most people who practice this way of work, people in different countries, people who speak vastly different languages, discover that in fact there is a language—more a way of speaking—born of this discipline itself, shared by those who practice it.

Sometimes movers surprise themselves and each other by spontaneous experiences, like the man dancing in this round, that perhaps occur in direct relationship to the development of a more accepting inner witness, coinciding with a developing trust in the presence of outer witnesses. Sometimes witnesses are surprised by a desire to become a mover because they want to do what he is doing, to enter the actual movement being made. *"I am the one who sees a woman walking just in front of each witness in the circle. I want to walk with her."* The experience of the original guideline of entering with no agenda begins to become more complex.

New guidelines appear when there is a conscious need for them expressed by a mover or a witness. Usually at this time in the collective process, questions of boundaries arise. People learn about a need for clarification of boundaries by speaking their experience and by listening to others speak theirs. When a mover's work challenges an agreed-upon guideline for the collective, discussions regarding safety become necessary. The growing freedom to move as one must becomes inextricably bound to the felt presence of each participant. Here movers cannot do whatever they need to do. Here they can only do what they need to do if they can do it with their eyes closed and simultaneously maintain awareness of and respect for the presence of the other movers and witnesses.

Because I cannot know what other witnesses or movers are feeling during a long circle, I must rely on my own experience of safety as a witness to guide my sense of responsibility as leader of the collective. When I feel unsafe I ring the bell and end the round. It is not safe for a mover to remain in a merged state with his inner witness for any length of time. Such an extended absence of presence can also make the moving body and the witness circle an unsafe place. For example, it is not safe or appropriate for a mover to express rage in the circle, as rage is an experience in which a person is merged with, overwhelmed by, sensations and emotions. Raging means losing connection with the inner witness. Anger can be safely explored when a mover can express the sound or energy of his experience and simultaneously stay in relationship to his own material and to others around him.

Movers often fear imposing their sounds on other movers and witnesses. Some sounds are agreeably too continuous, abrasive, shocking, or painful, but it is very hard for movers to anticipate the effect of most of their sounds on others. What is experienced as completely disruptive to one moving witness or witness might not even be heard by another. As the witness/teacher I encourage people, within an awareness of the potential impact on others, to intend to keep their sounds as close to direct expressions from the body as possible. Words, rather than raw sounds, can at times take a mover away from what he is experiencing, the premature meaning interfering with a committed engagement with sensation and emotion.

It is not safe or appropriate to purposefully sexually stimulate oneself or another. Because of the safety in boundaries, this particular guideline allows movers to open more to their authentic experience of their sexuality. Here the work is learning how to come into conscious relationship with the great and natural force of eros, including, at times, learning how to speak it. One blessing among many that can be received from this practice is the liberating work of distinguishing between sexual and sensual experience.

Another guideline emerging concerns the authenticity of the attention of the witness circle. Sometimes due to what a mover is experiencing or what a witness is experiencing or perhaps the relationship between the two, it can become too difficult for enough witnesses to stay present enough to ensure safety for the movers. When this happens the energy of the witness circle begins to waver. If the teacher or any witness feels unsafe, they can spread their arms wide to alert other witnesses that there is a need for more attentive connection. If the wavering continues, I will ring the bell to close the round. No matter how important any mover's work might be, if the witness circle is not in a conscious enough relationship to it, the circle is not a safe place for movers or witnesses. It is natural that there are times when the container "breaks." It must to have authentic strength, but then it must be mended. In this practice a call for more consciousness becomes the mending, empowering the circle, making it safe enough again to hold what moves inside.

Seasons pass. We are now meeting for a full day each time. Red tulips, their stems long and supple, stand in a glass vase on the low table. A woman quietly lights a candle before taking her place in the witness circle. I invite people to trust the integration of the phrase "I am the one who" as they move, as they witness, as they speak, as they listen. As we integrate an embodied knowing that we are part of a whole it is no longer necessary to speak it. Yet there continue to be times when using such a phrase in relationship to specific experience can be clarifying.

For an hour and a half the emptiness is filled and emptied, filled and emptied, again and again until the witnessing of the emptiness completes the ritual. During the transition, many now are exploring the writing process in relationship to embodiment. When we gather to speak and listen together some read instead of speak their experience, followed by a nonverbal signal that they have finished. In this round there are only three movers. When we gather afterward, one witness becomes a speaking narrator.

The braiding begins with the mover with the long gray hair.

> Hiding my face under my hair, I slam my feet
> down, dragging my body round and round. Angry
> phrases recite themselves over and over again in
> my mind. When I lie down the tears come. With
> the edges of my hands, I draw a barrier along the
> floor, marking a wall. Let no one enter. I feel an
> aversion to even the image of being touched. I
> become an island.

I hear a mover sobbing. As I remember my
own pain, I must track her cries.

The mover with the black shawl steps into the circle.

I am walking in my socks, walking backward,
wrapped forever in my shawl. My socks are peel-
ing off, like skin, like longing as old as skin, one
by the stone bowl, one farther away. I remember
another time of socklessness, when as I move with
cold feet I know I will never find my mother, that
I never have. No matter the fusion, the isolation.

I see the woman in the black shawl walking
backward, shedding her black socks.

The mover with the white shawl witnesses and then becomes a mover.

I see you and feel a despair—mine, yours,
hers, and theirs—as you walk backward
under the blackness of your shawl, as you
leave your socks behind. I name you as the
one who suffers. I name you as everywoman,
everyman. Wrapped in my own shawl . . .

I go to the stone bowl. I offer my neck to the
emptiness, arching my head back, feeling heat in
my throat. I am being moved. Folding my shawl,
leaving it in front of the bowl, I make an altar.
Turning back into the room, I leave the vessel in
search of your socks. I must find them.

I see the mover at the bowl ever so gently
make a white altar with her shawl, leave,
and begin a search for the socks.

I find one sock nearby and place it on the new
altar. I hear another mover crying, crying our
despair, crying our isolation. I must find the other
sock, bring it back and place it on the altar. I have
to find it.

I see the mover searching. I hear the other
mover crying and my belly tightens. I am
frightened. I look away. I want to leave the
room. I remember carrying my mother up the
stairs this morning. Confused and anxious,
she mutters and cries into my chest. I can't
bear it. Now I reach my arms out toward
the other witnesses for support, receive it, and
am able to stay.

My blind search intensifies. I have to find the
sock. Instead of a sock, I find feet. I know these
feet. They carry the woman who carries our
suffering under her black shawl. We become the
same as our foreheads touch, now our cheeks, our
arms, and our hands. I am you. You are me.

I see the mover who is searching for the sock
find the mover with the black shawl instead.
I see this moment. I need this moment.

You touch my feet and I know gratitude and grace beyond desire, beyond desire. I feel found beyond that old place where I feel lost.

> *I see two women, tender, together. I'm inside your spell. As a man, I feel the tragedy in my relationships with other men. I want such intimacy there.*

You within me now, I leave you, soon frantically searching for the other sock. I touch the mover who cries but she recoils. Swimming in the inconsolable cry of isolation, I become disoriented, even panicked. I can't find the sock and I don't know where I am! I surrender. Will someone take me to the empty bowl? Take me, please take me.

> *I see the mover frantically searching. I see her surrender. I hear her call for help. I see a woman leave the witness circle, take her to the bowl, and return to her own cushion.*

Still wrapped in my darkness, I slowly walk in search of the great bowl. Arriving, my feet touch something soft. Bending to touch it with my hands, I find my sock on a folded shawl. I place my other sock next to it, the one I had tucked into my pocket when I stumbled upon it a while ago.

> *I see the woman with the black shawl discover her black sock on the white altar at the bowl. I see her take her other black sock out of her pocket and place it on the altar.*

Left at the bowl by my escort, I take off my own sock, prepared to lay my own suffering next to yours on the altar. As I do this I find your other sock, the one I've been searching for!

> *I love seeing the face of the mover who has been searching for the other sock when she finds it on the altar, an awesome moment for me.*

We meet this time at the bowl as you gather the folded altar shawl and wrap me in it. I wrap you in mine.

> *I see an exchange simply occur, white shawl and black shawl pass hands, exchanging dark for light, exchanging light for dark, just like that.*

Slowly arriving back at my cushion with the black shawl around me, I open my eyes, in gratitude for the circle holding, in gratitude for finding you, for finding your socks, for receiving the black shawl, the essential black shawl.

Now another mover speaks.

I find your foot and hold on. Touching you, my crying finally stops. You rock me. In your foot, there is consolation.

> *I am so satisfied when the mover who is crying reaches out to the foot of the mover*

who shed her darkness, the one now stand-
ing in the white shawl. Oh the strength, I
imagine an invincible strength inhabiting
women's feet!

As the movers' inner witnesses strengthen, outer witnesses can begin to feel a shift from being present *for* the mover toward being present *with* the mover. Sometimes a witness experiences the whole moving body as more dominant than the individual bodies. Such witnessing can be experienced as a merged, dialogic or unitive state with the whole. Here the other man reads his collective witnessing, a story reflective of his dialogic experience.

I'm the one who witnesses an ancient tale
slowly unfold to the solemn music of a
woman weeping. This is a story about three
journeys, a great cauldron, and the miracles
that occur when we surrender to the truth of
not knowing.

Once upon a time, a woman under a black
shawl walks backward shedding her old
skin, first off of her right foot and then off of
her left foot, leaving her new skin still wet.

Another woman goes in search of these
skins. Finding one, she places it on an altar
that she makes with her white shawl near
the great cauldron. She then begins crawling
in search of the other skin, not knowing that
at the same time and not too far away, the
woman in the black shawl is stumbling upon
her other skin, stooping to pick it up and
putting it in her pocket.

*Instead of finding the skin, the woman who
searches finds the woman who shed her skin.
With great love she dries her still wet feet
with her hair. These two women become mirror
images of each other. Their movement of face,
hair, arms, hands and fingers are the same.*

*Soon they part. If both pieces of old skin are
not on the altar, healing will not occur. In
my mind, I speak to the woman still searching: "The skin is in the pocket of the one
who shed it." Not knowing and never finding it, she surrenders and calls for help. Now
she is escorted to the great cauldron.*

*Here she meets her own suffering. Here she
meets the woman who shed her skins. Here
the pain of isolation is soothed by connectedness, by touch and timing. Here transformation occurs as I imagine all of the socks in the
cauldron, burning the dark into light and the
light into dark.*

Another witness reads her offering, a poem reflecting her knowing of a unitive state with the whole.

*Black shawl
White shawl
Black sock on white altar
White sock
Black sock
Black sock on white shawl*

White hair in black hair
Black hair in white hair
Red petals red petals
Take me to the empty vessel
Gather me up
Breathe me in

Black heart white heart
Black opening black opening
Take me to the emptiness
Take me to the emptiness

Opening opening
Take me to the emptiness
Take me home.

○ As the work develops in a collective, when a symbol appears in an organic way for a mover, as it does in this group, often many others recognize it personally or as a part of a collective theme. Symbols can be forms in the mind and/or felt sensations in the body. If one allows the symbol to mentally guide or conceptually reorganize the experience, the symbol itself can interfere with a depth of conscious embodiment. However, within a natural timing, when an individual surrenders to a symbol, descends into and follows it, embodiment of a deeper truth can become a transforming experience. In this situation, for the woman with the white shawl the socks begin as symbols of suffering but soon become a stimulus for direct experience as they lose their representational quality. When this occurs in synchrony with the experience of enough individuals in a group, spontaneous collective ritual can arise, as it does in this situation. Each mover's work becomes an offering. Each witness presence becomes an offering.

How do movers and witnesses know when to go to a mover and when not to go to a mover who is crying, like the woman in this round? Discernment practice for a moving or seated witness is complex when he experiences a mover's continuous cry. How does he feel in the presence of someone crying whom he might name as sad, hysterical, frustrated, or lonely? What kind of nearness or touch does he need with this mover? If he chooses to go to the mover, he could discover that the mover definitely does need someone to come and feels welcomed. Such a synchronistic outcome is a blessing. Or he could discover that he is interrupting the mover's experience by trying to be near, to soothe or to help him when that is not what the mover wants.

Identifying intuitive knowing as different from projection, judgment, or interpretation can be enormously helpful. There are times when a seated or moving witness intuitively knows that the mover who is crying needs someone to come. There are times when it is known by others that the mover is doing just what he must do alone, and therefore offering presence from where one is becomes another kind of synchronistic outcome, another blessing. Perhaps there were seated or moving witnesses in this last round who were not approaching the crying mover for such a reason. Acting from a place of truth, either in stillness or movement, can be a hopeful and generous response.

Sometimes a mover's inner work is stopped by the act of his crying. In this round the mover's crying does not stop her work. When a mover is crying, he has another opportunity to practice discernment. Does he want someone to come to him? If he doesn't can he be clear about his boundaries, as the mover in this round is: "I touch the mover who cries but she recoils."

If he does want contact and no one comes, can his inner witness manage his needs well enough? If he does want contact and someone approaches him, what kind of nearness or touch does he need, can he allow? At this time in the collective practice participants become more deeply engaged with

these questions concerning the relationship between pain and comfort, projection and intuition.

As intuition becomes a clearer guide in the moving and witnessing
experiences, participants shift into a way of talking to each other that
becomes more intimate. Because people begin to trust not only in their
developing ability to own their projections and judgments but trusting that
others also have strong enough inner witnesses to do the same, it becomes
appropriate for the pronoun *you* to enter the dialogue among people. Until
now, it has been important to follow the guidelines encouraging the for-
mality of "the mover" or "she" or "he," which was helpful in protecting
each individual from being not only named but addressed directly. As the
language becomes more intimate it often becomes more simple, more
truthful. At times the fewer the words, the deeper the relationship among
them. After so many years of practicing toward conscious speaking, the
birth of poetry, like the offering from the last witness, emerges into the collective experience.

The
Conscious
Body

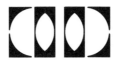

Offering

Tzu-kung asked, "What do you think of me?"

The Master said, "You are a vessel."

"What kind of vessel?"

"A sacrificial vessel."

CONFUCIUS

Emerging Forms

True perfection seems imperfect,
yet it is perfectly itself.
True fullness seems empty,
yet it is fully present.

True straightness seems crooked.
True wisdom seems foolish.
True art seems artless.

The Master allows things to happen.
She shapes events as they come.
She steps out of the way
and lets the Tao speak for itself.

TAO TE CHING

❏ Maturity in the practice of the discipline of Authentic Movement becomes manifest in the phenomenon of presence. It is not necessarily true that we are more present now as we step into the privilege of offering from the conscious body, but our ability to notice when we are present and when we are not has become heightened. When we are present, more than the details of personal history, engraved into the body matter, are evident.

Though the details never really change, because of an evolving practice toward growing consciousness, our relationship to them can change. This changing relationship occurs because of experience of being seen, seeing, belonging, of touching and being touched by others. A felt distinction between personality and presence becomes apparent as giving and receiving require less and less of the self. Presence allows offerings to emerge from the body as vessel. Within the open space of a witness circle, the discipline itself grounds the arrival of such offerings.

As individuals cultivate an inner witness with developing clarity and compassion I see them arriving, one by one, into a clearing, an open space. Here encountering another awakens a desire to make an offering and awakens a desire for the presence of another to receive it. Perhaps people have been seen enough by others. Perhaps they know that they belong enough. And when challenged by fear or awe, perhaps they remember the ineffable bright energy within and around themselves. As they acknowledge each other here, their movement and their words become offerings. Their presence becomes an offering. In this clearing, as longing pours into the practice of concentration, an experience of devotion becomes known.

Participants arrive and leave this clearing in silence, gathering in the studio for many full days, only talking together when engaged in the speaking and listening aspect of the practice or in evening seminars. They lodge and eat nearby, also in silence. This social silence frees people to stay focused inwardly, to release themselves from what is habitually understood as a social responsibility. In the absence of social discourse empty space exists between people—at meals, on the path to and from the studio, waiting on the lawn just beyond the wisteria. Witnessing one's relationship to such empty spaces, noticing the desire to rush in and fill them with words or noticing one's relief born of permission not to socially engage, helps bring more clarity into the experience of relationship. At this time in the work some individuals begin to crave not only silence but solitude, and create personal retreats in response to changes in their inner lives.

In conversations with me as the teacher, each person who is considering committing to the offering practice chooses one or more ways in which her unique gifts can be developed, guided by her individual aptitude and nature. Those eager to continue working with the relationship between body and word commit to a study and practice of the discipline of Authentic Movement and embodied text. Those wishing to bring their study and practice more fully toward the transformation of the gesture itself commit to the discipline of Authentic Movement and dance. Because the discipline is centrally concerned with a developing articulation of body and word, it is natural to witness offering circles filled with dance and poetry or prose. However, painting, drawing, sculpture, music, theater, and film sourced in authentic movement are also all potential realms of rich artistic exploration. And some individuals who are increasingly embodying in their practice an energy that is transpersonal in nature deepen their commitment to the discipliine of Authentic Movement, choosing this form to support their developing relationship to energetic phenomena. As such energy moves through the body it becomes an offering that can be witnessed and received.

Coming toward immersion in embodied text, dance, and energetic phenomena—and some choose all three—people are trusting their intention to be present, trusting that they can remember afterward what was happening when they moved, when they witnessed. Tracking becomes an automatic aspect of experience. "Where am I?" is less frequently the question. "Here I am" is more often known. Because the inner witness can stay present more consistently, people can surrender toward a deepening and widening of experience until new content, fear, or awe appear. Then it is essential to return again to the fundamental tracking.

It is here in the work with the conscious body that the study of intuitive knowing becomes more active. With full and continuing awareness of the possibility that what is thought to be intuitive knowing can in fact be projection, there is now more space for exploration of the phenomenon itself. Though always opening to the possibility of unresolved inner material interfering with clear seeing, at times in the long circles now people choose to shift their intention toward witnessing from a place of intuitive knowing.

Because of the mover's strengthening inner witness, developing directly in service of her own growth, it is less necessary for the outer witness to be in the service of the mover. Now the witness chooses to make offerings whether a mover whose work might be involved has spoken or not. It is no longer necessary to agree in the beginning on a certain number of designated witnesses in the long circle. In all aspects of the practice of offering from the conscious body, the mover and the witness increasingly manifest as the same within the circle.

The circle, one of the first forms known by men and women, is a shape within cultures that continues to hold the life of spirit. One can imagine movers and witnesses in original circles in which healing occurred as offerings to the gods were made. In the presence of a circle, poetry was sung, the full body was danced, other dimensions of awareness were entered. The spirit of the great and creative force was evident then and continues to be evident now within different mystical traditions in which prayers are embodied and spun into the numinous, emptying the self of that which is ready to be released, to be offered.

In the discipline of Authentic Movement, practice toward presence develops into moments when the body as vessel is experienced as empty. A longing to offer emerges from such emptiness. It is here that the form itself becomes transparent. Out of silence comes a word. Out of stillness comes a gesture. Out of presence comes a direct experience of energy. In the dyadic and collective body work, a prayer might be: "In your presence may I be able to embody my truth, speak my truth." Now, as offerings are made from an emptiness, from a place of experiencing the Divine in life in all worlds, a prayer might be: "In Your presence may light fill my truth in word, in gesture."

Embodied Text

The primary text of a mystic . . . is his human body. . . .

ANTONIO DE NICHOLAS

❏ Study and practice within the relationship between body and word develops toward experience with embodied text. Words that are seeded in the body knowing, birthed into consciousness and arriving into the world in a shape, named, and offered, can be expressions of devotion. When these words emerge from direct experience in the conscious body, out of a clear space, unencumbered by the density of specific personhood, they can become energy, illuminating a glimpse of the union between oneself and the Divine. The words themselves and the poetry, songs, and chants that they become in the moment of offering can be a direct knowing of the mysteries. Sometimes these words emanate this direct knowing when read by others outside of the text circle.

We begin with the long circle, standing instead of sitting. Experiencing the emptiness from a standing position allows the whole body to be moved by the literal force of it. One can feel pushed, pulled, rocked, or melted by opening into the emptiness. Moving in and out from witness to mover and mover to witness throughout the round of work can be changed by this shift in posture.

A ritual begins before the first round every morning, one that grew organically from the practice. From the standing position, after eye contact, the bell ringing, and witnessing the emptiness, someone steps in and walks counterclockwise around the inside of the circle with eyes open. Footsteps mark this space in this moment in all spaces, in all time. "Here I am. Here I am with you." Because people begin walking at different times, some are still standing while others pass in front of them. If either chooses, here is another opportunity for a different experience of eye contact between the one who is walking and the one who is standing.

Some choose to enter the ritual and those who do not remain standing as witnesses. People walk in their own way, at their own pace, until, acting from another place of discernment, they choose to either become a mover or to return to their place and stand as a witness. Here another way of initiating experience occurs as people choose to become movers or witnesses from an experience of walking rather than sitting or standing still.

The long circle opens, develops, and closes within an hour. In the second hour individuals write from their unique experiences as movers and witnesses. As people explore writing the embodied experience rather than writing about it, they can discover new ways of knowing the distance between experience and word, as well as the absence of such distance. The writing process brings a heightened awareness of words that emanate directly from the body.

The intention of the one who writes is to translate experience into words and/or to clarify experience to make it conscious, not to write poetry that is beautiful or awesome. If the words can be offered to others, genuinely received and accepted, experienced as nourishing or resonant, it is a blessing.

The practice of discernment continues throughout the writing experience. People write fluidly or thoughtfully, quickly or with pauses for tea, chocolate, and nuts. They hone and refine or never change a word. They write their own movement, their experience of another's, or that of the collective. When people's writing involves another, they consciously choose between: "I see a man" or "I see him" or "I see people" or "I see you," allowing the language to reflect the specific degree of intimacy that is experienced. Sometimes, when the pronoun *you* is chosen, they are addressing their God or the mysteries they enter.

In the third hour of any given round the work culminates in a seated circle in which embodied text is offered. In some ways, by becoming a reader one becomes a mover, and by listening one becomes a witness. As in the beginning of a long circle we begin the text circle by bringing our attention to the emptiness. It is out of the emptiness that words now appear. The one who has shared bends her torso forward, placing her hands flat on the floor, acknowledging the completion of her offering. Those who choose join this gesture, acknowledging that they have received what has been offered.

Though in certain moments of the text circle people continue to offer spontaneous spoken witnessing, an offering circle at this time in the practice is primarily a reading circle. Again, discernment is required. What does one choose to offer and when and how will it be offered? To whom is it being offered? If it is offered to a certain individual there is the choice to look at the person and, in very practiced groups, if it feels appropriate, even to say the person's name as the offering begins. Sometimes it is an offering to the whole group. If it is an offering to the Divine presence, the one who offers is encouraged to choose where to direct it: into the emptiness of the circle, down into the earth or up toward the heavens, or perhaps to the Divine presence within the person to whom the offering might refer.

Though the primary intention here is toward the practice of offering and receiving, individuals feel a deepening experience of being seen and of seeing as well as a greater experience of belonging, of participation in the whole. In the text circle words are first offered in the form of reading poems or prose. As the group work develops within this context, some of the words offered are echoed back by those who are listening. And later, as the relationship between body and word develops, the echoes become chants and songs.

The same six people who participated in the collective body work arrive today for a five-day silent retreat, each choosing to continue his or her work with the relationship between body and word. Though the birdhouse is empty this afternoon, we can hear one dove call from the persimmon tree. Someone points to the elegance of the white creature eating the exquisitely orange fruit.

It is time to begin the long circle. Standing, we no longer reach out to make the circle of bodies more visible, trusting our energetic presence. Eye contact, emptiness, circling the inside, some become movers, some become witnesses. I see movers crawling, rolling, reaching, sliding in and out of the two rectangles of light shining onto the floor through the big doors across the room. One man sits in stillness the entire time with a pool of light in front of him. After an hour has passed I ring the bell three times, and the long circle ends with our witnessing the emptiness.

People find places in which to settle for a time to write. One woman is using her folded shawl as a cushion, sitting on the window seat just inside the door. One man stretches his legs out on the grass, leaning against the tree at the end of the lawn. Two women are on the bench outside the door on the small deck and two other people gather cushions and sit near the stone bowl in the corner, one having brought the candle with her. I can see the light from the flame placed down in the center of the bowl.

Another hour passes and people return for the reading circle. From body to word to voicing from the body—one long braid is woven of poems and prose offered by movers, moving witnesses, and witnesses. A paradox emerges. The utter uniqueness of each voice is essential, evidence that the offering must be made to the collective by just this person. And just this person can become every person as the words are received, at times entered.

Now a mover begins by reading her experience.

> Entering the circle
> entering the mandala
> entering the womb
> held safely here
> nourished here
> I can live this strange
> and blessed body life
> belly, bones, lips
> tears, memories
> thought stream.
>
> Floor pulling feet
> through open spaces
> becoming pigeon-toed
> walking all bent in
> knees almost knocking
> ah, it feels so good
> to walk ajar
> walking into oneself
> instead of anywhere else.

Another mover reads.

> I walk the circle in tears
> I walk the circle in tears
> in time
> in song

I belong
forever
thank you
good enough
I am good enough

Two different witnesses respond to her reading.

> *The momentum of your walking*
> *holds the world up for me.*
> *I count on your walking.*
> *I count on your walking.*
>
> *You stir the room for me.*
> *You cry for me.*
> *I need you right here right here*
> *being what you do.*
> *Tracking your tears*
> *I map these tears.*
> *I name each one.*
> *Sorrow wells under my ribs.*

And another mover reads.

> the bowl   the empty cup
> fills with the world
> let it pour
> the cup fills with light and tears
> your deep sorrow and mine
> this light this neck this shimmer
> this fist of hardship I kiss it again
> one more time my little life of hardship

one more time this poor, tragic world
this bright shining world
pouring forth
one more time
let it pour.

A man responds first as a witness and then as a mover.

I see you kiss your fist of hardship
I kiss my own.

I stand breathing. Your tears propel me
into bearing my pain
of being a father
a father of a baby
who never stopped crying.
I hold her again.
May I bear the tension,
bear the confusion
the terror, the tears.
I hold a bundle
and rock back and forth
as long as it takes, as long as it takes.
I hold my baby again.
I see the Great Mother
holding me holding my baby
and peace comes
around my arms, into my heart.
I stand in awe
holding, holding
my baby.

Another mover reads.

> I go to the bowl
> I was a baby there
> abandoned
> long ago.
> I go to the bowl
> my legs vibrating so loudly
> I can barely hear
> my own breath.
> Slowly my arms pull around
> circling me down and into the well.
> Arching backward
> dipped again, my wrist dipped
> into the darkness
> so much dark radiance inside
> dark radiance so much dark radiance.

> *The altar of emptiness, I see you arriving there.*
> *I see you dip backward, stirring a bowl of light.*
> *I am witnessing. I am awakened.*
> *I am witnessing. I am meditating.*
> *The difference is my focus on you*
> *the you in me.*
> *I am meditating. I am witnessing.*
> *I never want to stop.*

Three different movers read.

> Reverent. I open my eyes and discover
> I have been a partner to something
> bigger than I am.

I cover my eyes seeking darkness.

I don't know if this is the moment to move or be still. I don't know if this is the time to witness or the time to keep walking. I don't know if this is the moment to turn to the left or to the right, to lift my shoulder a little, to move one finger or one thumb or one whole hand. Is this the moment to touch you? I cannot know. I move to the center.

> *I am suspended, as you turn to the right,*
> *lift your shoulder, move a finger and*
> *now your whole hand. Relieved, I see*
> *you move to the center as if you are*
> *floating, as if you are carried. I become*
> *weightless.*

Here a mover continues her reading from moments ago.

> I cover my eyes seeking darkness.
> Pelvis lifting inch by delicate inch
> inhaling
> my yoni receives the world
> lowering my pelvis inch by inch
> my yoni gives birth to the world.
> I tremble.
> I sing. You come
> and take my hands from my eyes
> take my hands in yours.

Your hands, soft and human
your hands hear my song.
My song sings itself.

A moving witness responds, followed by a witness.

Not knowing
not knowing what to do
I am wishing
wishing for someone
who can guide me.
When I move to the center
of the circle you appear
just as I imagined, on the floor
low and singing, singing
the song I deeply need.
I take your hands into mine
listening.

Without hesitation
I place my heart in your hands
feeling delicate layers of your
presence settle in me.
I recognize you.

Another mover reads.

What is my correct posture
for prayer? On my knees
I press my palms together
over my heart. No.
I place one hand

on top of my head
the other hand on my heart.
No.
Now with my palms facing out
my hands go out to the sides of me
and I arrive into my center.
Barely turning from side to side
I am receiving.
My prayer is energy received.
I am praying.
My prayer is energy directed.

This is the place for prayer.
I pray my secret prayer
for my husband, for myself, for us all.
This is the place for prayer.
Prayer fills my witnessing.
Forgive me. Do I really see you?
Forgive me.
I see prayer
in your walking the circle.
I see prayer
as you hold the baby.
I see prayer
when you dip your wrist into the bowl.
I see prayer
in your hands covering your eyes
prayer in her hands in yours.
I see prayer
as your hands come out to your sides.

Do I really see you?
Forgive me.
This is the place for prayer.

this last round on this last morning
it is the window to the outside that calls me
it is the fire within that calls me
balancing both worlds inside my body
how can I speak this last prayer
this poem is my prayer
I say the names of my loved ones into the bowl
I say the names of my loved ones into the bowl
a shadow passes over
a dark shadow of wounds, hurt, loss anger, sorrow
my life, my nature   there is nothing to fix
my life is a dark stone
my life is a white feather
may the emptiness bless us
may joy be strong
may we continue
may we continue
I hear your song.

Watching the wind move the flowers, I am sitting on the bench outside the studio door, waiting to greet participants for another retreat. People arrive in silence, two first, now one, now three. One woman is carrying a bouquet of cosmos, all white. I place them in a vase on the low table and we begin: eye contact, emptiness, walking the circle, witnessing and moving and then writing, translating experience from body to word.

As people prepare to read some of what they have written I describe a new way of participating that has organically evolved from the text circle practice. Words spoken by the ones who offer have begun to enter the listeners' responses, appearing in their offerings, creating echoes.

> Someone reads either their moving or witnessing experience. Besides responding with eye contact or with another reading that feels chronologically or contextually appropriate, I invite you as listeners to echo a word or phrase with which you resonate. This experience is distinctly different from the earlier work in which witness's responses to what movers say is in the service of the mover. I invite you now to echo specific words that are offered because, as you receive them, they feel as though they belong to you, because you are drawn to them.

A mover reads:

> Entering the circle
> entering the mandala
> entering the womb
> held safely here

As we are all listening to this mover read, if anyone hears a word or phrase that they recognize they can echo it back by using the exact words that were read, an opportunity to practice receiving what is offered.

Now a listener echoes:

> held safely here

Similarly another person echoes in recognition:

> held safely here

The one who offers or the one who listens can also echo a word or phrase over and over and over again, letting it change and develop. Here a listener echoes.

> held safely here
> I am held safely here
> I am safe here
> here I am, safely held
> here I am

Another listener now echoes in response to how the reading is changing.

> here I am
> here I am
> I need to be here

And another echoes his version, still changing the words to reflect his experience.

> I need to be here
> gratitude, gratitude
> may I stay
> may I stay

Sometimes many echo the same word or words of the reader.

> gratitude
>
> gratitude
>
> gratitude
>
> gratitude
>
> gratitude

As the inner witness clarifies in the echoing of words and sounds, the distinction between the mover and the witness becomes not only less clear but also less important. The original offering becomes released, transformed as the collective gives voice to that which has been received, recognized.

Movers and witnesses feel seen in unexpected ways even though the intention in choosing to echo is not to be in the service of the one who has read by repeating their words. At times, echoes are experienced as archetypal ripples of wisdom. The mover needs the witness. The witness needs the mover. The one who offers needs the one who receives. The one who receives needs the one who offers. Presence becomes possible because of the presence of another.

It is time to begin the text circle. We gather, witnessing the emptiness, not knowing what will arise.

> Rededicating myself to my fear I am the first to
> step into the empty circle, sheltered by my *tallit*.

Am I calling each of you in the witness circle to
join me in singing? Am I simply declaring, "I am
ready. Come when you are." I walk, clasping
myself. Tears, so many tears. Quietly I say the
Shema and now I sing.

I am ready

I am ready

Two different witnesses respond.

> *Round and round goes the song forever*
> *Eyes closed, lips trembling, face lifted*
> *My grandson's first cry*
> *The crone's endless wail*

the endless wail

> *you circle moaning*
> *stir the room stir the room*
> *with sound like a river*
> *stir the room*
> *drape the room*
> *river of sound*
> *drape the room*
> *river of sound*
> Shema, Shema
> *stir the room*

river of sound

Now a moving witness reads.

I enter it or does it enter me?
my hands, these hands, they touch
your moaning, your breathing, your cries
this earth pulls me down now
I lean back open mouthed air sucked in
blown back out I am empty empty and lit
I disappear here at the altar of my body
I am a mover dissolving
only hands only mouth only round dark sound
and light opening

opening I am not here at all
opening I am only here.

I enter it or does it enter me?

This earth pulls me down

and light opening

Now the one who offered the reading, after hearing echoes, responds by
repeating her own words again, this time in a new way, as if hearing her
words for the first time, grateful that they are being given back to her.

and light opening

and   light opening

and   light opening

Another mover reads.

Dragging my feet around the circle
my feet drag me deeper into the opening

the opening I remember.
I remember I am wearing the circle
an old opening.
I remember the opening of September
and yesterday's opening.
I remember: this is my work
opening.
I remember this again
and for the first time.
My head falls down.
My spine drops long.
Falling I remember
remembering hesitating trembling
I breathe a great tremor
discovering a nearness of you
in a tremor
a matched vibration
of hand and heel.
The nearness of you makes
something possible

                    this is my work opening

                    the nearness of you makes
                        something possible

A moving witness responds.

Trembling I stand very near you
facing you.
This is where I stand.
I don't know who you are

but I feel you in me.
This is where I stand.

I don't know who you are

This is where I stand.

Another mover reads.

Spiraling down through the earthbody
our threatened and vulnerable Earth
down through a whirlpool
headed right to the center
feeling air ripples, soul ripples
moving through my fingers
saturated
in sacred breath of nothing
generating everything
right here right here
here in my hands

A listener echoes and keeps going toward her own experience.

sacred breath of nothing
right here, here in my hands
here, I hold it
I hold my sacredness
my soul right here
I am here
I am sacred

A witness reads.

> *Your fingers, I see your fingers*
> *sifting through light*
> *sifting through life*
> *my life*
> *discovering my memories*
> *my lost places.*
> *You find them again for me*
> *sifting. I remember you.*

> > > *sifting*

> > > > *my lost places*

A mover reads.

> Listening to the wind outside
> I listen to the sounds inside
> here on my back, my hands cupping
> tight caves over my eyes.
> With my toes curled
> my foot reaches up
> an eye now in its sole
> a periscope seeing you.
> This eye, my eye, travels
> arrives in the palm of my hand
> now seeing my other eye
> in the palm of my other hand.
> My hands open, extend
> come closer

I see me seeing myself
through light
light between my hands.

Three different witnesses offer the same experience.

I see light between your hands.

I see light between your hands.

I see light between your hands.

Two different movers read and then the first one continues.

Seeing light in the empty vessel
I crawl to it
falling roundly down
into nothing
heading for silence.
longing for silence
for the ceaseless storying
to melt, to seep into silence.
While sounds of the circle
send me seeping
and falling
someone places her body
against the soles of my feet
as if I were living
as if I belonged. Stay.

I'm longing for silence

stay, stay near me, stay

Belonging
being who I am,
all of
who I am
for a long, long
time
in truth, for eternity
amidst us all
I am here.
It won't be long now
it could not be long
before I remember
it is my predilection
to belong.
It is yours in me.
Long be consciousness
long be compassion
long be
belonging

I am here being who I am,
all of who I am

before I remember

long be consciousness

before before

belonging

You stay
against the soles
of my feet
or is this God?
I hear:
"You are okay
I know your pain
I am with you
You are not alone."
Is this God?

                              Is this God?

                                 Is this God?

                                    I am with you.

A mover offers a final reading.

Entering one more time
minutes before the bell
going to my barrette
this one here
that I left in the space
when I became a witness again
forgetting.
I see it now.
I see that I have left
some part of me behind
that I no longer need.
Entering one more time
minutes before the bell

I lie down
slipping in
slipping my barrette
into my pocket
slipping
into the hushed
sea of silence
of delicate silky
light for a few precious minutes
my hair untied.

The cold winter rains have come again—more woolen socks, more candles, more hot tea. The paper white narcissus here on the table must be longing. Their stretch out into the space is magnificent. We begin by walking the circle, the sounds of the rain flooding into our silence. People move and witness, write and rest and prepare to participate in the gift of offering, in the gift of receiving.

As the offering circle is developing, echoes continue. Some people begin to gesture as they read. Sometimes people read a piece once, put down their journal and repeat their offering or a part of it over and over, gesturing as they speak. Sometimes echoes become chants or songs, some with accompanying gestures, some without. As the words come back into the gesture, back into the body, people are encouraged to explore a reentering or an entering for the first time in a new way. We are moving from body to word and back to body again but this time, because of a developing inner witness, we are arriving in a new place. We are arriving in a new place with gratitude as the distance between the moving self and the inner witness, between the body and the word, lessens.

It is scary to start, we begin.
Let freedom in
my body loosens
let it loosen
my body freedoming loosening
dare I obey it   dare I obey it
can I endure this freedom?
walk the circle, shake arms, shake arms
sit, stand
tiptoe and breathe
let light in
I am handling the light
the glint and glimmering
now it's here now it's gone
now it's here now it's gone
one moment!
one brilliant moment
my body freedoming loosening in water
Oh, I am rivering now
let it river
let energy come
let energy go
one minute here   next minute gone

the glimmer
the light
my body
let it loose

The reader keeps going.

the glimmer the light my body let it loose
the glimmer the light my body let it loose
the glimmer the light my body let it loose
the glimmer the light my body let it loose
the glimmer the light my body let it loose

Others join her in the rhythm of this chant, repeating it over and over, over
and over for a very long time, until it naturally completes itself. After a time
of silence the next person reads, opening her palms in front of her chest,
her hands pulsing in a rhythm that is synchronous with her words.

Grace
she enters me
through the palms of my hands.
I kiss that place
that knows to open
remembering
this is my only moment
right now, this my only body
my only fingers, my only toes.
This man near me
these eyes with me
this throbbing in me
all I have, all I am
exists just now.

> this my only body,
> this my only body
>
> all I have

A witness reads in relationship to a mover who hasn't chosen to read.

> *Over and over and over again*
> *your thumbs rubbing over each other*
> *comforting me*
> *soothing me*
> *over and over and over again*
> *I trust you to stay with the small motions*
> *for as long as the need lasts*
> *With you I treasure the small, ordinary miracles*

A mover reads.

> just now
> one drop from my left eye
> one drop from my right eye
> pooling
> in the hollow
> between my collar bones
>
> > *There is a cave behind*
> > *the little nook between*
> > *those two bones*
> > *way inside the secret domain*
> > *of your throat.*
> > *And I follow inside my cave*
> > *going for an inner meeting*
> > *with the warmest, most affectionate*
> > *Gods of my vulnerability.*

inside my cave

warmest, warmest, warmest

those two bones
those two bones

A listener echoes *"those two bones"* and now chants this phrase, placing his finger in *"the little nook between those two bones."* Others join the chant and some also join the gesture. Now I hear the three words being sung to the tune of a familiar rhyme, and as we all join in I see much smiling, I feel much joy. Slowly, as the song is sung over and over, opening toward what it is becoming, the lightness shifts toward a drone, the words easily changing from *"those two bones"* to *"my bones"* to *"home"* to *"come home,"* moving back into a chant and finally, as people's hands beat *"the little nook between those two bones,"* the words move from *"come home, come home"* into silence. Quiet and still for a while, the empty space opens toward another offering.

I have been afraid of feeling, of feeling too much. I ask for this: to feel. I want to feel everything—disappointment, dark shame, pure joy. I receive a dance and I dance it the best I can, though clumsy at times. But I am this dance. This dance is my gift. Can I give it away? I send the blessings out. My path of feeling leads me to you, to this circle, to this moment. It is not the perfect place for me. It is the only place right now, here where I am. I am not the perfect person to be here. I am here.

I am afraid of feeling too much

I am afraid of being too much!

I am not the perfect person

I am not perfect

I am not perfect

I am here flaming
a fire flapping my shawl raising my arms
breathing my fire
my body is a flame
my wrists hold torches
up is down light is dark in is out
words burn up with breath
past language
past anyone who's there who cares
where is the word
here is the fire

> *You flap and rise*
> *I lower my hands*
> *onto the floor*
> *grounding my heat*
> *grounding my vibration*
> *grounding my fire.*

Another mover offers.

> Heels pounding, rhythm rising
> head thrown back
> my mouth an open circle
> I dance in the fire.

I dance on the fire.
I am the fire.
I am ecstatic.
My heart is beating wildly.
My heart is beating wildly.
I am on fire.
My heart is beating wildly.
My heart is beating wildly.
I am big energy.
I am big energy.

> *Big*
> *wild*
> *fire, wild fire*
> *burns my spine*
> *burns*
> *as I see you*
> *dance*
> *as I receive*
> *your light*
> *marking space*
> *marking space*

The same reader continues to offer more after hearing a listener's experience, perhaps encouraged by feeling seen, received.

> Can I contain it?
> Does it contain me?
> I am in the energy.

The energy is in me.
I am inside the Divine.
The Divine is in me.
My heart is beating wildly.
My heart is beating wildly.
My heart is beating wildly.
I am on fire.
I can't look now
and I can't say.
My heart is beating wildly.
Returning to my place
I hear an inner voice:
"Come home
Come home."

                    I am on fire

                        can I contain it?

                          I can't say

                          I can't look

                              come home
                              come home

"Come home, come home." We hear these words, already brought into this collective field, now whispered many, many times until two people are whispering them together as they slowly move toward each other into the center of the offering circle. The intensity develops in eye contact and in the whispered voices until a more grounded chant appears. Now, instead of staying in the middle, each person keeps scooting on her knees across to the other side of the circle, exchanging places. The chant moves back into a whisper and finally back into silence, stillness. A long time passes and another mover speaks, her voice trembling.

> Shaking and trembling
> quaking and shaking
> no words
> no feelings
> I don't know.
> Spinning to the floor
> on the edge of the circle
> waiting
> no answers
> I don't know.

> I don't know

> I don't know

> I don't know

> *We sit in the circle*
> *our bodies around you.*
> *I see you. I feel you.*
> *I hold you, not knowing.*

Sitting
prayers in a circle
prayers
in your eyes, the palms of your hands
the soles of your feet
touch faces, touch spines
we are holding
the living spirit
its many altars in our flesh
great mother church.

we are holding the living spirit

I am giving up everything
to be at the altar of this moment
I am sacrificing shame and fear
and am I enough
to be at the altar of this moment
I am letting go
    letting go of the place at your throat
      where the tears pool
    letting go of the gift of your dance
    letting go of the flapping of your shawl
    letting go of your heels pounding
    letting go of your shaking and quaking
    letting go in order to be
      at the altar of this moment

I am letting go, letting go, letting go

Bowing deeply to the circle
and all who have moved in it
a great honor
to touch its smooth expanse
to flow over it like water
to smoothe and rake it
the Zen temple garden.

Dance

There is an energy behind all occurrences and
material things for which it is almost impossible
to find a name. A hidden, forgotten landscape
lies there, the land of silence, the realm of the soul,
and in the centre of this land stands the swinging
temple . . . in which all sorrows and joys, all
sufferings and dangers, all struggles and deliverances
meet and move together. The ever-changing swinging
temple, which is built of dances, of dances which
are prayers, is the temple of the future. . . .
We are all one, and what is at stake is the
universal soul out of which and for which
we have to create.

RUDOLF LABAN

◖ The discipline of Authentic Movement springs from both ancient and modern dance. Reaching back through the lives of modern dancers, past the lives of ballet dancers, past the times and cultures in which the dancer performed ceremony, we arrive at a time when being and dancing were inseparable. The history of dance tells us of women and men's great and natural, original desire to dance in the circle, to dance the fullness of the cycles of life, regardless of place or time, culture or speech, regardless of the name of God. In such times, prayer is the body dancing. Dances of suffering become dances of healing. Dances for and with the gods become dances because of the gods. Whole in this one circle in the presence of each other, the embodiment of spirit heals. Here the roots of the discipline of Authentic Movement are each evident: healing practices, dance, and mysticism.

As dance grew from a worshipful expression of the collective body in ritual toward the Western expression of the individual body in performance, fewer people danced. As the development of the discipline of Authentic Movement evolved into the collective body work, more people began to dance again, sometimes in new ways, with more consciousness, more freedom. Whether movers are being still, moving, or dancing, at times witnesses can feel like an audience. Questions emerge concerning the relationship between the experience of being a performer and being a mover, of being in an audience and being a witness. Both performers and movers wish to be seen. Both audiences and witnesses desire to see.

As the inner witness strengthens, movers can feel a difference between an experience of being looked at and being seen. Those who perform can feel a shift toward mover consciousness as they work in relationship to their audiences. Witnesses can feel a difference between an experience of looking at and seeing. When experiencing themselves as an audience they can feel a shift toward witness consciousness as they come into relationship with the performers. Here, as offerings are made within the dance circle, there are moments for individuals, and sometimes for an entire group, when there is no separation between the one who dances and the one who sees the dance.

An experience of mystical dance emerges in this discipline out of gestures discovered within authentic movement. The dances are mystical for the movers and for the witnesses when the energy of the movement is emerging from direct experience in the conscious body. Emptying the gestures of the self, movement mysteriously can become sacred dance.

The same six people arrive for a five-day silent retreat to begin a study of the relationship between the discipline of Authentic Movement and dance. We pick apples from the trees here in the orchard, bring them into the studio, and peel and core them, filling the empty vessel with seeds and skin, stems and leaves. We talk about the new ways in which the practice is developing, ways of working that have been organically growing out of moving and witnessing in the long circle.

We begin with a long circle, with standing, making eye contact, witnessing the emptiness and walking around the inside of the circle, choosing or not to connect with those still standing. Some continue as movers, others become witnesses. In this format standing is again the primary witness posture, with sitting as an option. The long circle is followed by a brief transition in which people note or draw specific gestures that they find compelling, their own or another's. Gestures are not named. The inner experience of gesture is not named. Instead gestures are consciously reentered and allowed to develop.

The dance circle also begins and continues with everyone standing. After people make eye contact the bell rings and the emptiness is witnessed. Preparing to make an offering, someone enters the emptiness with her eyes open! She is reentering her own gesture, discovered as a mover or, for the first time, she is entering another mover's gesture, discovered in her witnessing. During a complete offering circle individuals can offer one or more gestures or none at all. A gesture is chosen by a mover or a witness not because it is interesting, beautiful, or powerful. It is chosen because the one choosing deeply recognizes it, needs it, must know it. Here an individual becomes aware of a specific movement and then chooses to enter it just as listeners in the text circle become aware of a specific word or phrase and then echo it.

Now I speak of the new guidelines.

When you make an offering, choose where in the space to start: near the edge or in the center, facing in or facing out? Does the gesture originate from a standing or kneeling position or with the full body on the floor? Take time in entering this shape, this breath, this gesture. If it is another's, practice receiving it just as it was offered, changing nothing at this time of first entering it. As you repeat it over and over it becomes yours. Choosing a gesture of your own or another's that can be easily repeated works better in this format because the repetition, the rhythm, become a natural guide toward entering it.

Because your eyes will be open as you enter this gesture, your inner witness will have a different relationship to it. Here you are invited to not only focus on your movement but, while doing so, to stay connected to witnesses in a new way. If the gesture is not yours, a witness might realize that it is her gesture from the long circle and thus could be experiencing another way of being seen.

Other witnesses might remember seeing this gesture that a mover made in the long circle and are seeing it again in a new context in the dance circle. Perhaps they never saw it because it was being discovered when they themselves were moving.

In the dance circle, often one or more of the witnesses will see this offering, know it as one to be entered, and, following their own timing, choose to come into the circle. Like the one who first made the offering, the witness becoming mover will choose where in the space she wants to be and at what level in space: standing, lying, kneeling, sitting. Each one can choose to enter with thoughtful placement in relationship to the circle. Each one can practice receiving and entering the gesture exactly as it was offered.

Repeatedly embodying a gesture invites its natural development. As movers continue to repeat it the now-collective gesture begins to subliminally change, not from an idea about making it more interesting or exciting or more one's own, but from an organic place within the movement itself. How can the mover find her authentic movement from this developing gesture, with her eyes open?

Witnesses who don't choose to enter a particular gesture remain as standing witnesses. Because now the original offering is transforming into other offerings, at any moment a specific gesture could call to a witness to enter. Standing as witness makes a seamless transition into movement even more possible. Just as in the circle where text is offered, soon individuals lose track of who was the original mover, who was the original witness. Within any particular collection of movers in the presence of any particular collection of witnesses, when the individual work becomes synchronous with the whole, dance can occur.

It is time to begin the dance circle. Because of the way the light falls, as we stand in a circle I notice shadows of each person across the room from me glowing along the inner edge of the space that our bodies are outlining. We acknowledge each other, I ring the bell, and we now directly focus on the emptiness.

As the dance circle opens:

> *I see a woman step into the center and, standing in stillness for a moment, slowly lift her arms straight up above her head, flex her wrists, tilt her head back, and on an*

exhale softly sound: "Hah." Lift, flex, tilt, exhale. Lift,
flex, tilt, exhale. Lift, flex, tilt, exhale. Another person
steps in, standing directly behind the first woman, and
slowly lifting her arms straight up above her head, flexes
her wrists, tilts her head back, and on an exhale softly
sounds: "Hah." Now a third person enters, standing
behind the second person, doing exactly what the other
two are doing.

Though the extending of their arms, the tilting of their heads, and the
sounding are all happening at different times, the gestures and sounds flow
together as if of only one moving form. Three people standing in a line are
making this same gesture over and over, this time not changing it at all, until
it completes itself and they return to their witness places. The circle is
empty again, waiting for the next offering.

I witness a woman now who witnessed throughout the long circle earlier
and continues to witness so far in this offering circle.

Her inner witness:

I see a man step into the center offering a gesture that I
recognize from the long circle. Bending his knees, widen-
ing his stance, he slowly lowers his head toward his
chest. His arms scoop long and down, his hands cupping
nothing as he now lifts them up toward his face. With
wide empty spaces between his fingers, the palms of his
hands turn toward each other and now, with flexed
wrists, he pushes his hands away, straight out in front of
himself. Keeping his arms straight, he lessens the space
between his fingers as his two thumbs become straight,
extended toward each other, their tips now touching.
Straightening his legs, this mover looks into the eyes of a

*witness across from him, framing her face with this form
that his hands and thumbs are making.*

*I see him take a deep breath and, stepping to his right,
he repeats the gesture, bending his knees, dropping his
head, reaching down with his hands and then cupping
them as they come up. His hands, creating the form as
he straightens his legs, push his arms straight out in
front as he looks into the eyes of another witness, framing her face with his hands. Again and again, each time
taking a deep breath, bending, stepping, scooping, cupping, pushing, he gazes into the eyes of another witness.*

*I see a woman step into the circle to the left of this man.
She makes these gestures exactly in rhythm with the
man who continues this offering. As her arms straighten,
her hands form a frame through which she looks into the
eyes of still another witness. Two movers now are doing
this gesture series in synchrony. Imperceptibly, as the
woman steps to the right with a bent knee, I see a little
hop. This little hop into each moving phrase mysteriously
appears in the man's stepping to his right, and soon
both are taking this gesture to the side into bigger and
bigger leaps.*

*A third mover leaps into the circle, standing to the left of
the woman, joining what now is a dance, with audible
breath, in torsos rising, in arms shooting up above the
heads as movers push off the left foot, the right one
stretching up and to the side.*

*As exhales become shouts another mover enters. The
dynamics increase and each time the series completes*

itself in a pause, punctuated by eye contact with wit-
nesses and now with other movers. The dance builds into
larger and larger movements as the first man who makes
this offering spins back into his witness place. I see three
movers all developing the same movements simultane-
ously, eyes flashing, until the leaps and the swings, the
shouts and the flings, become smaller, more quiet, and
each returns to his or her witness place, leaving the circle
empty again.

I also see this gesture in the earlier long circle when the man is in the corner behind the stone bowl, bending his knees and scooping up above the
bowl, now "looking" right through the form his hands are making as his
arms push straight ahead. I am on my witness cushion diagonally across the
room from him, feeling as though he is "looking" right at me even though
his eyes are closed. I feel seen.

In this same long circle I see a woman witnessing him, focusing on his work.
I see the lines in her face soften, her shoulders drop, her feet slightly moving her body from side to side. A small smile appears on her face. Maybe she
is becoming a mover. As I witness her later in the dance circle stepping in,
joining his movement, I notice a small smile appearing on my face, my feet
moving, as if I am becoming a mover. The original offering continues to
transform. The mover and the witness visibly become the same.

◖ In this particular dance the relationship between the mover and the
witness has dramatically changed, not only because the mover's eyes are
open but because the dance is repeatedly punctuated with specific eye contact between the mover and the witness. After years of the mover's inward
focus, energy now extends outward directly toward the presence of the witness, who for years has been extending energy toward the mover. Now

energy consciously meets energy. This dance especially marks a significant developmental step in the practice of the discipline.

In the dance circle, the inner witness for each person is continually challenged because of working in a collective body. When the energy builds, as it does in this round, sometimes witnesses feel pulled in by the momentum itself but do not feel a call to enter, do not consciously choose to enter. A tension can arise for witnesses especially when many movers are dancing right here, within this circle, so close and intimate. "Am I a witness or am I a mover?" There are times when witnesses experience this choice, this call toward more consciousness, as very painful, challenging their sense of personal boundary. Feeling the swelling of energy, of movement expanding, wanting to belong, realizing one could be swept away—an opportunity arises to make a conscious choice and to experience the outcome. Here the danger of merging rather than staying in a dialogic relationship to the moving collective body becomes obvious, reminding us of the social and political implications of such choices we might or might not make in the world.

Another challenging place of discernment, germane to the tension just described, appears when a mover, whether the one who made the original offering or not, no longer feels authentically connected to the current movement. At times it is difficult to recognize this and then to leave the circle and return to one's witness place. One aspect of the ground for these kind of choices is laid in earlier work when moving witnesses choose to make contact, sustain contact, and end contact.

In the dance circle the intention is to stay authentically connected to everyone in the room and simultaneously to stay connected to inner impulse. When first entering a gesture sometimes it is tempting to close one's eyes because of what now is a deeply familiar way of working with emerging movement. Sometimes two movers, maybe because their eyes are open, can become locked into the intensity of doing the same gesture together over and over and quickly lose awareness of the other movers and/or the circle of witnesses, interrupting the rhythm of the collective work.

Sometimes the one who is making the offering needs time to fully embody the gesture. When she is in transition toward allowing it to become her own, there are times when the offering is not yet clear enough to be recognized by others as a movement to be joined. Similarly, when another mover or others join and are in transition, extended patience and continued focus for both the movers and the witnesses are required in support of enduring moments of a felt dys-synchrony. Some gestures from the long circle are offered, most are not. A mover can notice her inner experience when a specific gesture, perhaps very important to her in the long circle, is not offered by a witness. Sometimes a person will make an offering and no one else joins. Inner work can become necessary to remember that a gesture not offered or joined does not necessarily mean that the gesture was not seen, received, or appreciated.

In my morning walk before we begin I see the glistening detail of each thread of three spider webs. They are impeccably whole and imperfect, stretched between the branches of the rock roses. As people appear on the brick path, preparing for another silent retreat, I am keenly aware of our impeccable wholeness which, like the webs, includes our imperfections.

It is time to begin. We follow the ritual of the long circle with the ritual of a dance circle.

I see one woman step in, her gaze downward, her eyes open. She places the toes of her right foot to her right side, pushes her body around to her left, and steps down on her left foot. Repeating this gesture, this rhythm, she begins to turn and turn and turn in one place. I see her turning, spinning, dancing a circle. I remember her turning earlier today in the long circle. I am relieved now to see this one gesture describe the empty space around her, as concentration forms in my body. She spins, her hands lifting her shawl up behind her. She spins and I hear one witness singing a wordless, joyful song, a song full of light. She spins and I see the gaze of every witness riveted on her dance.

Now I see two other witnesses lift their shawls up behind themselves, as if joining her but from their stationary places. She spins and spins until the song and the dance complete themselves and she returns to her place, leaving the emptiness filled with crystalline impressions. We witness the emptiness.

Now I see a woman, in her place, begin to sway slightly, forward and back, forward and back.

Her inner witness:

> I am being pulled into the circle to make an offering from my own movement in the long circle. As I realize this is happening I notice my heart beating fast and my palms are sweating. Here I go. I'm in now, leaving my place near the bowl. Walking across the room to the carpet's

edge, I turn and face back into the circle. I bend
down on my knees, placing the palms of my
hands over my face, though my eyes are open and
I can see through the light places between my
fingers. I rock down and over my knees and back
up again. I am rocking alone for a long time.
I see a woman come and kneel in front of me,
facing me, placing her hands over her face and
rocking her torso down toward the floor and up,
down and up.

I see another woman come and stand next to her,
facing in my direction, placing her hands over her
face and rocking her torso down toward the floor
and up, down and up.

I see another woman come and stand, facing me,
on the other side of the first woman. She is rocking her torso down toward the floor and up, down
and up. Her hands cover her face. We are rocking
together. I exhale deeply, audibly. I hear a witness
make the same sound. I am heard. I respond this
time with more sound. The witness continues to
respond to my call, and I respond to his until a
low lamentation emerges. Other movers are
sounding this sad cadence now in monotone,
this sad cadence: "uhmm ahmee ah   mo."

Now I hear all witnesses making this sound and
I can see their bodies slightly rocking forward and
back, standing in their witness places. As movers
and as witnesses, we are crying. Pulling my hands

down from my face and now pressing my palms
together, I see the mover standing in front of me
doing the same thing. Am I following her or is she
following me?

All movers standing now, the rocking becomes
bowing. I step into a walking, bowing gesture and
see that now three other women are doing the
same. We are walking. We are bowing. Walking and
bowing, walking and bowing, we come into the
center of the circle, forming a smaller circle.
Bowing with others, I am honoring the suffering
of others, honoring my own. I am not alone in
my grieving the endless suffering of our world.

All movers, all witnesses are droning: "uhmm
ahmee ah   mo."

Somehow, at some time, we walk and bow until
we each return to our witness place, emptying the
circle once again, once again, preparing it for the
fullness of what is becoming.

○ Earlier in the long circle this woman goes to her knees and rocks with
her face covered by her hands, weeping. This gesture is only hers in this
moment. Like any other personal gesture, it has the potential for becoming
archetypal. In the long circle a specific witness sees the mover rocking and
recognizes it as her own. In such a moment a witness can feel seen by the
mover. Now in the dance circle this same witness has an opportunity to
actually embody this gesture by entering the circle, becoming a mover as
she joins the gesture, finding it to be her own, perhaps participating in its

becoming universal. When each can stay in clear enough relationship to her own inner witness and not merge with the unfolding collective, such an embodied boundary strengthens the potential for authentic transformation of the gesture, perhaps transformation of the ones moving and of the ones witnessing.

Sometimes a person, when witnessing another person embody a gesture that was originally hers, sees her own gesture taken to places that she was not ready to go or afraid to go, yet yearning to go. Now seeing the other person moving into such a place because of her gesture, she might feel inspired, supported, maybe able to see herself a little more clearly. Because of the developmental nature of this work, it is rare that someone who feels ready to commit to the dance circle has the opposite response of not wanting to see her own gesture developed by another person.

The dance circle invites an investigation of new boundaries in the development of witness consciousness. Witnesses discover more opportunities for discernment. Beginning from stillness, if impulse suggests, a witness opens toward moving in place, intending to support, not interrupt, the witness circle or the moving body. Such movements can lead a witness into actually choosing to become a mover. In the individual and collective body work witnesses have been silent. Now witnesses are invited to sound from their place, sounding in ways that do not interrupt their concentration or that of others in the witness circle or the moving body. What sounds organically come while witnessing? What sounds can a witness risk making that would support, deepen, develop the work in the moving body? In this last round while a witness sees movers rocking, he echoes a mover's exhale and, following the development of this sound, he hears himself chanting: "uhmm ahmee ah   mo" and voices it.

His inner witness:

> As I witness, I am praying
> As I pray, I am chanting
> As I chant
> I rock forward and back
> forward and back
> I am praying
> for our poor and suffering world

We are working in the studio at night as we sometimes do while in retreat. I hear the owl early in the evening, a constant witness to our nighttime longing. A candle is lit on the low table, one on the corner of my desk, and one on the window seat, their flames reflecting, multiplying in all of the surrounding windows. The stone bowl is full of darkness.

After the long circle and a brief transition we begin the dance circle. In a long circle earlier today I saw a despairing woman pounding on the floor with her fist, demanding: "YOU BE MY MOTHER!" Pounding and slapping the floor, she continued insisting until the quality of her voice and her movement shifted into a plaintive plea, then into a whisper: "Please be my mother."

Now in the dance circle I see her offering this gesture as she lies on her belly, calling into the earth, hitting the floor as she calls: "mother mother mother." I see a man enter the dance circle and lie down on his belly with his head almost touching the head of the mover who is offering this gesture. Both bodies stretch out, their feet near the edge of the witness circle. He joins the call, his face into the floor: "mother mother mother."

His inner witness:

> I am here. I begin to roll from side to side with
> my head falling back. This time, facing her, I see
> her eyes seeing mine as she does the same. We are
> softly saying: "mother mother mother." Now I am
> touching the top of her head as she touches mine:
> "mother." Now I touch a witness's foot: "mother."
> I see this witness become a mover, touching the
> other mover's leg: "mother." As we look into the
> eyes of the one we touch we are saying this word
> together: "mother."

> That witness becomes a mover, touching the
> other mover's hair: "mother." All witnesses now
> are movers. All movers are witnesses. We are
> standing, kneeling, walking, reaching, touching
> each other, seeing each other, saying exactly
> together: "mother." The pace quickens, touching,
> seeing, saying: "mother." Who is it? Who touches
> his own heart first? We are all touching our own
> hearts, looking into each other's eyes, saying:
> "mother."

> I am my own mother, birthing myself, because of
> you. Seeing, being seen, we chant "mother mother

mother" as our steps become clear, as we reach for
each other's hands, as we spin into silence, into a
wide sweeping circle. Our heads are thrown back.
I know we are the same, you and I, you and I.
Here I am. I am here. Here I am with you. I am
ecstatic. I am whole.

⟦⟧ Here as the witness/teacher I choose to become a mover, to dance, see,
know the circle, move as one with the circle. I see the circle spinning.
Spinning, I am the circle. In the dancing circles there are times like this when
everyone experiences a unitive state with the collective. There are times
when every person simultaneously knows a direct experience of the whole.

As dance is organically discovered within the collective, the evolution
of the discipline becomes apparent in a multitude of ways. Each commitment toward being seen, seeing, participating, and offering, can be experienced as complete within itself, and simultaneously each place of work
prepares movers and witnesses for the next and natural transition.

In the beginning of the dyadic work, five minutes of moving can feel
surprisingly long because movers are just opening to the experience of conscious embodiment. Later, as the collective body work develops, movers wish
for hours and hours of movement time. Often it can feel as if there never is
enough movement time. And now the long circles in the embodied text and
dance work often last less than an hour as people become practiced in dropping more quickly into and emerging from a deeper level of experience.

In the beginning of the individual work, repetition becomes a potent
force within the embodiment of movement patterns. Here in the dance circle movers source their gesture with a repetitive movement. In the beginning of individual work, movers embody the gesture again to remember it,
to bring it into consciousness. Here in the dance circle movers consciously
embody the gesture to offer it to the collective.

Throughout the practice, until the dance circle, movers work with eyes closed. Sometimes, in order to clarify their speaking afterward, some movers close their eyes while reentering the movement. When moving witnesses become outer witnesses, first silent and then speaking, they shift from experiencing the other mover in the room with their eyes closed to experiencing the other with eyes open. Here, as movers and witnesses offer gestures to the collective body, their eyes are open.

In the individual or collective body work, when a mover suddenly opens her eyes, it is a way of responding to fear, disorientation, not enough internalized safety. When this happens, the mover is guided to honor this way of knowing, and to return to closed eyes only when it feels safe. Now as gestures are offered and danced, eyes opening expresses a longing to see, with these eyes open, oneself moving. There is a longing to see the others moving and to see the witnesses seeing. There is a longing to see the whole and simultaneously each part all at once while staying in conscious relationship to all that is arising within and around oneself.

Early in the practice a mover begins as the only mover and with no agenda. As the form develops into the dance circle, years of committed practice bring an individual out from her own movement and into another's. In the beginning of individual work the mover is discovering her own idiosyncratic gestures as they are forming in impeccably correct ways in relationship to the development of her inner witness. A mover can feel ambivalent about seeing her own gestures being made by her witness when her witness is speaking. Here as offerings are made, the inner witness can see herself well enough and therefore she does not feel invaded by what might have felt like imitation of her work by the witness years ago. Now many of her gestures can be given away, offered up, because they become integrated and no longer belong just to her. Once offered they belong to everyone.

Until now practice and study have centered on the relationship between embodiment and word. Here, trusting embodied consciousness enough, movers and witnesses commit to working with an absence of words, creating a new space in which offerings can be made directly from the body. Until now witnesses commit to sitting still, containing their experiences. Now witnesses come into the circle, becoming movers, alone or with others.

Offerings unfold into new gestures. New gestures are witnessed and become possible choices for new offerings that originate now in the dance circle, not before in the long circle. And finally, dance circles are no longer preceded by long circles. Gestures from the past, gestures new from this offering circle, and gestures never made before in any long circle, in any dance circle, appear for the first time, are offered, received, developed and danced. It is a blessing, a moment of grace, when a direct or unitive experience with others happens in one's presence. By the end of this most recent round there are no witnesses. In the dance circle, for the first time in the development of the discipline, there are times when everyone can become a mover because each one experiences a strong and present enough inner witness so that an outer witness is not necessary.

Energetic Phenomena

*The mind becomes empty and there is
an experience of being a witness in the body.*

AJIT MOOKERJEE

◖◗ Direct experience is at the core of energetic phenomena. Within the
discipline of Authentic Movement, direct experience is known as a unitive
phenomenon, occurring when the inner witness becomes clear, silent
awareness, when the felt separation between the moving self and the more
familiar experience of the inner witness dissolves. There is an awareness of
and immersion in the ineffable experience of nonduality. This definition is
similar to the descriptions of direct experience in the mystical traditions
derived from monotheistic religions, and of samadhi in Buddhism. A direct
reunion with soul, such experience of energetic phenomena can be understood as experience of spirit in both a concentrated and an expansive way.
Like spirit, this transpersonal energy has always been and will always be part
of human experience.

But in the Western world, until recently, too often spirit has been sacrificed along with the body in many religious traditions. As energetic phenomena becomes more visible in the West we can be reminded from
non-Western cultures that conscious embodiment of such energy is natural, deeply contributing to experience of wholeness. We can learn ways of

understanding this energy from the study and language of ancient and contemporary mystical traditions. Sanskrit, the ancient language of the subcontinent of India, is especially available to the West at this time when we are discovering an absence of words in our own languages, an absence of trust and deep understanding of such experiences. We have not grown up witnessing people experiencing energetic phenomena, held by the presence of a circle of elders. Because of few models, little understanding, fear, and judgment within our cultural history, our bodies, our psyches are not well prepared for such experiences.

Energetic phenomena is emerging spontaneously for many individuals within the practice of the discipline of Authentic Movement. Because this is a Western practice, grounded in the development of embodied personal consciousness, such experience is not the goal. Because the mover and witness begin each time not knowing, with no intention beyond the longing toward presence, such experience is not sought. If energetic phenomena manifests within childhood or begins to appear within the course of an adult life or appears specifically within an embodied awareness practice such as the discipline of Authentic Movement, our task is to receive it in gratitude and to learn how to come into conscious relationship to such a blessing. It is the development of the inner witness that makes this possible.

Though experience of energetic phenomena can occur gently or not so gently at any time in the evolution of this discipline, extensive practice in the dyadic and collective body work can help to ground and prepare the body and psyche for it. With such grounding practice it is more likely that the mover will not merge with the energy but instead consciously witness it. When energetic phenomena occurs within early individual work, as the witness/teacher I honor the presence of the energy by directing the person's attention toward practice in tracking it in relationship to physical movement and inner experience. Without continuing attention, especially in the early dyadic work, toward unresolved aspects of personal history, safe and clear work with energy can often be impeded. Paradoxically, because the energy can be a source for clear seeing, at times it can mysteriously be in the service of resolving experience mired in unconscious psychological complexes.

When energetic phenomena occurs within the collective body work, as the witness/teacher I welcome such experiences if the mover can stay in conscious relationship to the experiences and simultaneously to others in the group. There are times when individual work becomes more appropriate than group work. When a mover becomes ungrounded in her experience of energetic phenomena because of unresolved personal growth issues, individual work is necessary. If a mover is in a group and the energy for any reason begins to dominate her work and thus interferes with the work of others, individual work becomes useful. Sometimes individuals need to bring their attention completely to the gifts and challenges of the energy itself and its effect on their lives, thus choosing to work alone with a witness/teacher.

The commitment required for individual work at this time is the same as the commitment of the mover in the dyadic work: practicing toward staying present, tracking all that is arising and simultaneously practicing toward developing a conscious relationship to it. Yet when the energy is active, at times staying present can feel too difficult. Relating to what is happening can feel impossible. Movers can identify with the energy, with the content that arises. They can resist it, feel afraid of it, desire it, attach to it, feel confused or overwhelmed by it. Both inflation and deflation are natural and challenging responses. The presence of the witness/teacher becomes vital in support of such work.

An intelligence is experienced within this impersonal force, which demands, requires an awesome respect. Each mover experiencing energetic phenomena has a specific way of expressing or containing it, responding from the uniqueness of her nervous system. Some experience a raw energy, with no image or sound to organize it. Some receive visions, hear sounds, words, or clear teachings. Some enter other times and places, including the realms of the dead. Some experience extrasensory perception, psychic phenomena, or at times visitations or possessions by other entities. Many know both the formless and the formed ways of experiencing the energy. Each journey is distinctively different than all others, and there is great comfort in discovering strong and basic similarities among such initiating phenomena.

If individuals experiencing energetic phenomena don't already have a strongly intuitive nature, and many do, transpersonal energy heightens experience of intuitive knowing. For a mover this way of knowing can be manifest in an experience of feeling as though one is "being moved," taken, penetrated, rearranged, infused. These qualities of sensation are experienced without the density of emotion or thought, though such qualities can be followed by the fullness of personality in response. In a moment of direct experience, the mover can become empty.

For a witness this way of knowing can be manifest in an experience of clear seeing, seeing without the density of emotion or thought, increasingly at times without awareness of specific sensation. The witness can become empty in moments of direct experience. There are times when the mover knows when moving and the witness knows in witnessing that they are in a unitive state. Here the quality of experience for each is specific, imbued with timeless and infinite space.

For both mover and witness, direct experience occurs when the inner witness is only conscious presence. As the energy both concentrates within and moves through the conscious body it becomes an offering to the mover, to the witness, and, in an energetic sense, to that which is beyond us, that which we call our world.

Waiting this evening at summer's end, I am watching the dogs on the hillside roaming through the prickly grasses, recently scythed, still golden. The
tall man arrives with peaches cradled in the cup of his shirt. We leave them
lined up on the bench outside the door and come into the studio, settling
near the low table on our cushions. The intensity of his inner experiences
in the dance group led him to discussions with me concerning his wish for
individual work. I light the candle as he makes eye contact and moves into
the space, working for ten minutes. I call his name and he opens his eyes,
looks at me and returns to his cushion. Now he speaks his experience.

> I walk to the center of the room. My arms leave my sides
> and arrive away from my body, palms out. I am standing,
> waiting for direction. My right foot leaves the floor,
> moves slowly forward, and arrives once more on the floor.
> Standing, I am waiting for more direction. My palms leave
> the outer positions and arrive together in front of my
> face, move down over my face and torso and wait for fur-
> ther direction. My left foot leaves the floor, moves forward
> and arrives. My right foot leaves and arrives. I am waiting.
> I leave the center, arrive at the window, and wait. I am
> seeing that the way of the inevitable is paved with leav-
> ings and arrivals, with stillness and movement. So simple.

This kind of inner witnessing is a blessing. The edges of the pools become
more subtle, liquid, and disappear. He is not only tracking his movement
and inner experience seamlessly—his inner witness is becoming a more
vivid and loving presence. Because of his clear shift from personality into

presence, as his witness today it is unnecessary for me to offer him anything other than my presence. May my presence be enough.

The tall man arrives for continuing individual work but the evening hour is now dark as the seasons have moved. He lights the candle, speaking with me about how these new experiences of presence are affecting his life at home, at work. Though he tells me of an increasing worry about his responsibility in terms of his work because of deep exhaustion, he speaks of more peace within himself. He also speaks of an absence of an old and familiar armoring in relationship to his growing sensitivity to disorder, traffic, television, and conflict. He feels a particular kind of vulnerability emanating from his experience of a deepening presence within. He is gratefully glimpsing a new experience of strength that he begins to associate with this vulnerability.

Walking to the center, he turns and makes eye contact and closes his eyes.

His inner witness:

> I stand and wait for direction, becoming a
> boundariless field of pixillating vibrations. My
> upper torso suddenly jerks. I hear a high-pitched
> sound in my head. The vibrations become louder
> in my spine and neck. My neck tilts to the left,
> my fingers become locked in specific shapes. My

lower back aches. My stomach feels flat, pushed
back against my spine. I feel another sudden jerk,
this time more in my shoulders.

I feel my body floating upward. My feet are
becoming unwieldy, huge and itchy. I feel as if I
am not breathing. I would like to walk out of this
now but I can't. I am lashed to this spot but without ropes or emotions. I am not paralyzed, but I
am not able to actually move. I feel another jerk.
This is where I cannot see myself. I am leaving
my body. I open my eyes, in gratitude for the
presence of my outer witness.

My inner witness:

May my presence be enough.

After twenty minutes of work I see this man very, very slowly begin to
make the long walk back to his cushion. Here he tells me of his experience,
again with clarity and patience. He speaks of his willingness to surrender to
these sensations. We talk about what he describes as sudden jerks in his body
when he moves, which he has begun to notice in the last month. I tell him
the Sanskrit name for this phenomenon, *kriya*. Kriyas are spontaneous, automatic movements that can occur anywhere in the body. Though often
experienced as sudden jerks, they can also be vibratory or smooth. We also
discuss the phenomenon of his fingers extended into certain forms in relationship to each other. The Sanskrit name for this full shape of the hand
gesture is *mudra*.

We speak at length about the moment in which he becomes aware that he
can no longer consciously stay in his body and the moment when he
intends toward a return and the moment when he opens his eyes. Now his

practice becomes focused on such moments. What precedes these moments? What is he doing right before he realizes he is leaving his body? What happens as he is leaving his body? Because the content is new, because he is experiencing awe and some fear, effortful tracking—just as he practiced in the individual and collective body work—becomes essential again. He must commit toward remaining in his body consciousness while he is experiencing other ways of seeing and knowing, no matter how strong the pull is to leave, no matter how awesome the experience that calls him away.

I prepare the space for the tall man by sweeping the floor and lighting a candle. There is a knock on the door and I gesture to him to come in as I walk toward him. He makes it clear that he does not want to speak now and goes immediately into the work. I see him walk to the carpet, look at me, and close his eyes. He works for thirty minutes.

His inner witness:

> This space has become sacred for me because of
> sacred experiences that I know here. Standing at
> the edge, I brush off the bottom of my right foot
> with my left hand. Now I brush off the bottom
> of my left foot with my right hand just as I do

before entering the enclosed garden behind the
temple. Entering my sanctuary, my body becomes
an antenna. I vibrate. The kriyas come and go.
I see myself clearly here. Empty, I know clear,
silent awareness.

As I float up and get smaller I hear a song inside
my head as though I am singing it, but I don't
know this song. I have never heard it before. It's a
tragically beautiful song in minor key. This song
transports me more deeply into the vibrations.
This is real, really happening to me.

Cautious, I can't see as clearly now but I am not
ready to leave and I must come down. I don't
want to open my eyes to do it. I will myself down
by focusing my inner gaze on a tiny and bare
winter tree that I see, illuminated by snow, white
everywhere. I know I must return, open my eyes.
More kriyas. The ache in my back becomes terri-
ble. I am nauseated and weak. My stomach is
churning. My feet are burning.

Now, focusing on coming down, I'm being
painfully, aggressively shoved back into my body.
Arriving on the floor, I lie for a long time flat on
my back, my hands on my stomach. No one will
believe me. Can I believe me? I open my eyes.

We make eye contact as he turns toward me. We see each other here for an
extended time. When he crawls back to his cushion there is more eye contact. Because of the depth and duration of his practice, my verbal witnessing
becomes less necessary. At times in such a situation, the details of the expe-

rience of the witness can actually clutter the energetic field. Increasingly the witness becomes clear, silent awareness in the presence of energetic phenomena. My presence becomes my offering. My prayer is my longing: *May my presence be enough.*

◲ I do, however, participate fully in dialogue as the witness/teacher in responding to how the mover comes into relationship with his experiences, with his emotions and thoughts in response to what is happening. The tall man wants so badly to sing me the song he hears during his experience and cannot. He wants so badly to describe his experience. He says he is clear when he is there and knows exactly what's happening, though he feels now he cannot articulate this experience well. And when he tries to articulate it he feels not only frustrated but as if he is betraying the experience. When he doesn't try to articulate it or somehow bring it into form he can feel painfully alienated and, at times, less human.

Because of the extraordinary quality of direct experience, sometimes even with such developing clarity, a mover's mind questions if he is making up something, imagining it, or somehow creating it. Exploring the tension between doubt—"No one will believe me. Can I believe me?"—and belief—"This is real, really happening to me"—often leads to a deeper acceptance of what he knows to be true. He knows this experience is real because of his conscious experience of sensation that accompanies his movement.

The tall man can increasingly stay in his body while these experiences occur. Now he includes in his work the task of enduring what at first can be a very challenging transition back into a more grounded embodiment. This can be demanding, exhausting, not only because he must choose to contain the energy rather than open to it but because he is in fact moving from one energetic field into another. Such a changing within space and time becomes easier as practice develops. The rigor of practice is required as he learns how to experience other dimensions of reality while maintaining a witness presence.

In this discipline we continue to discover that mover and witness, moving self and inner witness, individual body and collective body, body and word are all at first experienced as separate phenomena and then known in moments of grace to be the same. Usually energetic phenomena is first experienced as separate from ordinary consciousness. With committed embodied practice it is possible to discover that ordinary and extraordinary experiences can exist in an integrated way.

The woman in the red socks has chosen individual work because of a developing intensity in her experiences of energetic phenomena in the embodied text group. She arrives today under an ominous sky, speaking of her relief in being here alone and some excitement about this choice.

We begin with eye contact. Closing her eyes, she walks to the bowl and slowly kneels in front of it. She delicately dips her fingers in as if there were water there. I see her bring her hand back to touch her third eye, her throat, and then the place of her womb. Soon she stands, making sweeping circles with her arms and hands over the bowl. After moving for twenty minutes she opens her eyes and looks at me for a long time before walking across the floor back to her cushion. She says she is not ready to speak about her experience and chooses to write.

After a time of silent transition, she reads to me:

> There is a wind inside
> a slate-colored wind
> a movement in swirls
> swelling
> sweeping across
> my inner landscape
> changing me.
>
> My upper body swirls
> little circles as I stand
> here at the bowl
> my feet tethered under me.
>
> I am lightly stroking
> the outside edges
> of my arms.
> I have no skin
> or maybe my skin
> is permeable.
>
> I know no separation
> between the inside of me
> and all that is outside.
> I am knowing my boundaries.
> I have no boundaries.
>
> My left hand arrives
> in the nook
> where my collarbones
> meet. My fingertips
> flame as they surround

a ruby
in the center place.
Now in my fingers
of fire
the ruby carves
my boundaries.
I have no boundaries.

Dissolving but still here
I don't know
if my eyes are open
or closed.
I see with my cells
as my head goes back.
Here is a being
a rapturous entity
the radiance of two arms
embracing me, a kiss
on my forehead
igniting me.
This I know.
This I know.

After she reads to me we talk together about the sensations of her boundaries changing and her feelings of safety in these discoveries. She speaks at
length about her deepening humility. She describes her inner witness as an
increasingly constant and compassionate presence. She experiences less
interruption of this presence from fear, doubt, and judgment: "This I
know." Except in acknowledging her gratitude she does not speak more
about finding the ruby under her chin. Aspects of transpersonal experiences, just like aspects of personal experiences, require containment until
it feels correct to talk about them. Instead she talks about the developing

sensitivity in her fingertips. She speaks of a moment in her home when she experienced much energy in her throat and, without thinking, placed her own hand on her neck. She was surprised to find that the pain and constriction relaxed immediately. She tells me of her experiences of heightened psychic perception. Sometimes she doubts this way of knowing when it arises out of or is connected to an experience of fear.

◻ One way of understanding the experience of constriction in this woman's throat is within the phenomenon called *kundalini,* a Sanskrit word describing primal energy. As the energy rises or falls in the body it passes through seven energetic centers called *chakras.* When the energy cannot pass easily through a chakra intense physical and emotional pain can be experienced, as well as unusual and expansive experiences of consciousness.

Energetic phenomena creates an economy of movements. For this reason, and because conscious time quickly recedes into a timeless space when entering or being entered by the energy, actual movement time for individuals working with transpersonal energy is usually not very long. This woman rarely works for more than twenty minutes now. As the inner witness strengthens in relationship to energetic phenomena, at times the mover can extend her formal practice outside of the studio work, without an outer witness.

The woman in the red socks returns weekly for many months. We speak together about her increasing inability to digest many foods, the new complexities in her intimate relationships, and her growing need for more naps in the daytime. Sleep at night is often interrupted by the energy, by visions. We discuss her experience of visions, which sometimes accompany the energy surges. These images, unlike visual fantasies, appear with a vivid presence, made of vibratory light, the energy itself carving them in minute detail. This woman considers her visions to be teachers, most of them offering wisdom, insight, and moments of transcendence.

An awareness of death consistently surrounds her experiences of visions, as well as other manifestations of her experience of energetic phenomena. She is coming into relationship with death by experiencing other realms of consciousness in other places, in other times. She says she is no longer so afraid of death but instead feels an intimacy or knowledge about its profoundly natural place in the cycles of life. She speaks of an awareness of all fear in her life being sourced in a fear of death. She tells me of a peace inside not known before regarding her experience of her stillborn son so many years ago.

Today, after lighting a candle and making eye contact, she walks a circle on the movement floor, pausing at each of the four directions. She arrives into the center and sits down.

Her inner witness:

> I am sitting on dirt.
> A fire burns nearby.
> People wander around me.
> I smell the dust.

I taste it.
All colors are muted
by it.

I take off my socks
in preparation
for an offering.
I am the one to be offered.

I stand up and carry
my beloved red socks
to the empty vessel
and place them inside.
Gratitude for all the years
of protection
because of these socks.
I no longer need them.

Returning to the center place
I lie down on my back.
My hands float down
across my face.
Light explodes into light.
Energy funnels directly
into my heart.
My heart becomes
enormous.
I become my heart.

I contract, all of me.
I am tension held.
I contract, all of me.
I am tension held.

Here at the center
the four directions converge.
I am my heart.
I am my heart.

I receive the ruby
with my left hand.
I pierce my heart
with the ruby
My heart is sacrificed.

My head is pulled
forward onto my chest.
I am seeing with one eye
in the center of my head
a clear lake.
Now immersed in the water
I am surrounded by
tiny and electric
blue, intricate lines
a highly ordered
pattern.
I am not surrounded by
infinity.
I am infinity.
I am clear, silent awareness.

In the beginning of this round I witness this woman place her red socks
into the stone bowl, remembering the day she placed her dead baby there.
When she returns to the center of her circle and lies down I experience a
shift in the light in the room. When I see her pierce her heart, I stand up
and remain standing until she stands and walks back to her cushion. As we
engage in eye contact I see the edges of her head becoming light, becom-

ing formless. She speaks moments of her direct experience, places of no duality, of no separation between her moving self and her inner witness. She speaks of holding these experiences in awe rather than in explanation.

The woman without the red socks arrives for continued work. Today we begin by sitting together at the stone bowl. As she sprinkles some ashes into the emptiness there, she tells me in detail of a ritual that she did at home in which she burned her red socks. She speaks of her life now as a series of rituals—making the bed, cooking, watering the plants, bathing. She tells me of new space experienced inside and around her. Her boundaries are suddenly clearer when she is out in the world. She speaks of a new voice of clarity emanating from herself. The voice of her inner witness and her speaking voice begin to be the same—more clear, more concise, more free.

Today she does not move until we come near the end of our time together because there is so much she choses to say about the changes in her life. Now she leaves our intimate and shared space at the bowl slowly and slithers out into the empty room, looking back for eye contact. Smiling, she waves to me with her right hand as she closes her eyes.

Her inner witness:

I go to the row of windows
standing at this end

where the lilac grows
outside here.
Opening my eyes
I see the tiny new buds.
Closing my eyes
and turning the lever
with my right hand
I roll this window
out.

One step to my left
and I turn the lever
and roll out the next one.
Another step
another window opening
another one
and another one.

I step to my left
and open one more
window
one more
and one more.

Outside, inside
pressing
the palms of my hands
together
touching my fingertips
to my lips I look down
down into the earth.

I see my childhood
bedroom, the pale blues
the soft apricot spread.
Turning, I choose
the sleeping porch
just above the sea.
I choose the pines
the empty sky.

The woman with the white shawl has been working with me in individual sessions for many months, focusing on the challenges of her experience of energetic phenomena. Today she speaks of physical pain and fear. As it becomes time for her to move she tells me of more fear, fear that feels potentially overwhelming to her.

We speak together about a necessary respect for fear. Fear can be a wise protection against opening to experience for which we are not ready. Trusting the inner witness to know when to surrender and when to bring one's will and say "no" becomes critical. She decides to move now, remembering that she can choose to stop moving and open her eyes at any moment.

We make eye contact and she reluctantly steps onto the wooden floor, walking directly to the bowl. Melting down into a crouched position, her toes tuck under her feet. She begins to rock forward and back, forward and back, forward and back. I hear her exhale getting louder and louder as she bangs back down onto her heels, her wrists pressed into the floor in front of her. Now and for a long time I hear her screaming. I see her slamming both hands in front of her onto the floor over and over again. Now she lunges forward, her hands striking out into the space in front of her. Her hands grab each other, clutch her face, her hair, her feet, now claw at her chest. Suddenly she crawls to the corner of the room and there I see her shaking, shuddering. I hear her whimpering. Now she reaches her right hand up to the plaster wall, tapping her fingers along the surface until they follow the wall down, landing on the floor, now landing on her foot. These fingers tap her foot until she becomes quiet. A long time passes and she crawls back to her cushion here next to me on the carpet.

While she rests I prepare tea and fill a bowl of hot apple sauce in the kitchen. When I return with the tray we begin to speak together. She expresses shock in realizing that, after all of the inner work that she has done, there is still a remnant from her infant trauma, a significant and surprising remnant. She speaks of a recent outpatient surgical procedure followed by deep pain and fear, which have continued. Now the pain and fear are gone. In the past she worked with deep focus and integrity as a mover in releasing energy from her infant trauma in the hospital, especially aware of the psychological wounding from the premature separation. However the specific pain and terror embedded in her nervous system because of mistreatment there never surfaced in her movement or witnessing work until now, following the medical procedure.

Today she relives the mistreatment. She speaks of a relief in letting such darkness into and through her body, a relief that a potent force which was previously invisible is now embodied, more visible and more conscious. She speaks of the tapping movement along the wall and how she knows it is not her gesture. As she surrenders to it she sees a small child standing next to her crib, his hand reaching through the slats and onto her foot, comforting her.

◯ It is not uncommon for unresolved aspects of personal history to appear even when so much inner work has been done, even when much of life is experienced as consciously unencumbered by the density of past experiences. Perhaps because of the maturity of this woman's practice, perhaps because of the presence of energetic phenomena in her life, the darkness and pain of this particular event passes more quickly than, for example, the darkness and pain discovered years ago when she first relived her experience of abandonment when she was an infant. Now she needs time for rest and recovery in response to the sudden plunge into fear and pain. Many months pass as these experiences integrate, as our work continues.

The woman with the white shawl comes today with warm bread from the bakery at the bottom of the hill. Sharing bread and hot tea we speak of her increased experience of energetic phenomena, which has seriously challenged her professional work and her ability to be in the world as she was before the energy entered her life. Her daily practice in this form has become her work. The energy at times now is experienced as stronger than her personal will, fiercely challenging her inner witness toward staying present. She chooses to come twice a week to strengthen her ability to stay grounded. I offer her very specific instructions, reminding her of a practice that she knows well but one that presently feels too difficult.

to keep your eyes open now as we are speaking. It
perative. If they begin to close you and I can walk
gether with our eyes open. Walking and physical
touch can be grounding.

When it is time for you to move, step into the space and find
your way. When you are ready, choose to make eye contact
with me and then choose to close your eyes. As you now choose
to open to the energy more directly, allow it to enter you only
if you can stay present, tracking all that is occurring within
you. The minute you realize that you are being pulled away by
the energy, open your eyes. When you do this I will come and
sit next to you and you can tell me with as much detail as possible
what has just occurred within you.

We begin as she lights a candle. I see this woman crawl to the carpet's edge
and, sitting on her heels, gaze into the emptiness. She is doing this for a long
time. Now she stands and walks a circle three times, counterclockwise. She
stops at the bowl and, bending down there, she places her hands on the rim.
She gazes into the emptiness for a long time. I see her stand again, circle the
room three times, and walk to the center, turning to make eye contact with
me. I see her seeing me for a very long time. Now she closes her eyes and
bends down to the floor, landing on her side, her hands near her mouth.
She moves for three minutes and sits up, opening her eyes. I go to her, ready
to listen. Working hard to keep her eyes open, she speaks to me very slowly.

> I lie on my side.
> One leg is crossed
> over the other.
> Energy comes into me
> rising up through my foot
> the one on the bottom.

My torso curves
forward
as my hands
my wrists, extend
pushing into my belly.
Undulations
undulations.

Great sounds
erupt out of me
as my torso arches
backward.
Will I explode?
May I be able
to let it through.

My wrists press
into me and now
straight up above me
as my head falls back.
I am undulating into
nowhere
and
this is where
I cannot see myself.
The energy is too big.
I open my eyes.
I sit up.
I look at you.

She asks: "How do I hold even this?" I ask questions, one by one, and we find the answers together: "How exactly do you come down to the floor? On which side are you lying? What sensations do you experience as the energy enters your foot and rises up into your legs and torso? How far up does it rise? When do your hands leave your face and come to your belly? What is the sensation of sound surging through you? Where do you feel it? Do you experience any emotion in response to what is happening?" Because the force of the energy challenges her wish to stay present, we must track every aspect of this experience in support of her inner witness being able to stay present. This is the only way I know to "hold even this"—with consciousness.

I stay nearby and witness her choosing to close her eyes again, opening to the energy. Each time she makes the same movements: walking the circle three times, stopping at the bowl, coming to the center, bending to the floor, lying on her side, and her foot begins to move. Each time she intends to open her eyes the minute she realizes that she is no longer present, choosing to deepen her commitment to a tedious and arduous practice.

Time passes as this woman commits to a daily practice in her home in which she works just as she does here with me except that she writes when she opens her eyes, writing everything that she can remember about the time in which her eyes are closed. She tells me that even at home the same series of gestures, in the specific order, are repeated each time. She names this particular work her ritual.

There are times when this woman comes back to her cushion, too exhausted or not able to track. She asks me to tell her everything I have just seen her doing. As I accompany her again within the work of the beginning practice I am awed by the larger cycles of repetition, by the curves in the spiral, the mystery of return. And I am reminded that in returning she is arriving into a familiar place but with a different consciousness. Some days she can stay present while moving for five or ten minutes, other days only one or two. Slowly the time lengthens, and she begins to feel that she is coming into a dialogic relationship with the energy rather than merging with it. This is the work.

◯ Because this woman has extensively studied and practiced the discipline of Authentic Movement she is deeply familiar with an intention toward presence. Years ago, in her beginning practice in this discipline, just months before she discovered her wrists pressing into the floor as a part of reliving her infant trauma, she experienced a moment in which her moving self and her inner witness were experienced as the same, an experience of union. This first appearance of this specific gesture occurred within a fleeting, transpersonal moment.

> "It is as though my arm is being lifted, being
> moved. And my wrist is hot, full of tiny vibrations.
> I cannot describe this very well. . . there is no
> time, no space suddenly in this moment. I am
> whole here."

This experience was soon followed by the extension and pressing down of her wrists onto the floor, becoming an active part of a repeated series of gestures concerning her infant trauma.

> "With my back arched, I rock backward onto my
> heels and now forward toward that pressing place,
> my wrists pressing, held down, tied down. I am
> tied down at my wrists."

As her work developed in the collective body format she continued to experience this specific gesture in many different contexts. In her work in the embodied text group there was a time when she read:

> "my body is a flame
> my wrists hold torches."

Here she is entering direct experience, but this time with a much stronger inner witness. Most recently, when she was extremely challenged to stay present as the energy surged through her body, the flexing and pressing of her wrists gave shape to the inexhaustible force.

> "My torso curves
> forward
> as my hands
> my wrists extend
> pushing into my belly.
>
> My wrists press
> into me and now
> straight up above me
> as my head falls back."

It is not uncommon for a gesture that forms within a body memory of a trauma to become the gesture which marks a gateway into transpersonal experiences. It is not uncommon for flexed wrists as well as specific and extended placement of fingers to be a significant part of the experience of energetic phenomena.

The woman with the white shawl now knows that during her infant trauma she experienced other realms, ones she entered in the absence of her mother, in the presence of mistreatment. But she entered those realms with no inner witness. Now she commits toward strengthening her inner witness in relationship to the energy moving in her body so that she can stay conscious of what her body is doing as she enters other realms of consciousness. In her practice she moves from feeling at the mercy of such a force into staying present with it for as long as forty-five minutes. As her inner witness stays, the energy integrates, developing a consciousness that can ground awareness and that, by its very nature, can continue to assist in healing the trauma.

Time passes. Today the woman with the white shawl reports her pleasure in surviving such a tenacious grip on her being. She is managing more of a constant flow of the energy without disrupting her still simplified daily life. She no longer repeats her beginning ritual and instead is entering new movements. She speaks of less tension, less effort, more fluidity. She speaks of a subtle sensation of vibration in her spine while we are talking together. She speaks of infinite space around her while we are talking together.

Today she is remembering when she first relived her infant trauma. In that experience she entered a specific place in which time and space disappeared. "I am locked into this particular sensation, and elongated, narrow, and perilous place which I totally fill." Now, years later, at times she knows no boundaries as she enters an eternal vastness, a deathless place within which all life radiates. Now, as she looks beyond the window seat at the delicacy of the violets in the garden, she speaks of a recent experience in which she feels pierced by the unbearable beauty of a wild rose growing in the dunes along the edge of the sea.

Still sitting on our cushions, we are seeing each other's eyes as an hour passes. Eye contact becomes a longer, deeper experience of communication, another way of knowing ourselves and each other. I witness her end our eye contact and walk to the carpet's edge. She bows to the space and walks in. She comes down onto her knees, placing her hands on the floor in front of her. Diving under one arm she lands on her back, her arms down at her side. I see that her hands and arms are moving toward her head, yet I cannot see them actually move.

Her inner witness:

Lying on the floor
on my back
with unbearable longing
I slowly pull my hair
out and away from my head
with just my fingers and thumbs.
I am pulling a part of me
I am pulling me
to the edges of me
now beyond
the edges of me.
Letting go, my hands
open. Heat burns
in my palms.

Now my fingers
on top of my head
separate my hair
making a portal.
Is it my yoni opening
or the crown of my head
opening?

I am being pushed through.
I am pushing through
a second birth.
I become born
from my own body
into new consciousness.
I become born.

Time passes
and I stand up
pulling my shawl
around my shoulders.
I bow to the space
as my departure
creates
emptiness once again.

This woman speaks with great gratitude about her experience of energy as a remarkable gift. In the home of a new friend recently she is astounded to discover pictures of a sculpture from an ancient culture in which a woman is dancing with her arms raised, her wrists extended, her hands in flame like torches. What was once only her gesture now within her own awareness becomes a universal gesture.

◻ As a mover's relationship to transpersonal energy becomes conscious enough, the mover expresses interest in working as a member of a small group with others who are experiencing similar phenomena. There is a longing to hear others speak of such experiences. There is also a desire to explore energetic experience that might occur while witnessing another person move who is embodying energetic phenomena. Here, in some ways, the process of evolution through the development of the discipline is repeated, with individual work preceding work in a collective body. However, as the density of personal history becomes less of a dominating force, new blessings are received, new challenges are addressed as movers and witnesses encounter new ways of knowing. Honing the preciousness of the development of human consciousness, individuals circle through longings to be seen and to see, to participate and to offer, each time moving toward that which cannot yet be known because of committed practice grounded in what can be known, an experience of conscious embodiment.

The woman with the white shawl has been continuing to work with me here. As her daily practice strengthens, space and time continue to open in the studio and in her life, the differences between these two worlds becoming smaller. Coming here now in this early evening light, we notice that the colors outside the studio and the colors inside are remarkably the same. After we make eye contact I see her walk to the stone bowl, to the emptiness within it, source of all that is. Closing her eyes, she stands for a long time, now flexing her wrists, her palms facing down, over the vessel, as if she is warming them by a fire below.

Her inner witness:

> Coming nearer and nearer
> to myself
> discovering no self
> a soft infusion
> I am pure being.
> I am clear silent awareness
> here for all time
> here for no time
> here, not here.
> I stay here
> becoming.
> My gratitude rises
> spilling over
> into no words
> here where I am.
> When I leave here

I will stop
at the market
and choose
some pecans.
Pecan pie
for giving thanks
gratitude indescribable.
Here.
Clear silent awareness
here, now not here.
Thanksgiving.

She opens her eyes after moving. We see each other and she returns to her cushion. With a radiant smile she tells me her plans for Thanksgiving, what she will cook and who will be there. She tells me about her cat having kittens in the laundry room, about her evening walks. It is time for her to go now into this dark evening. I turn on the lights that shine along the brick path. Good-bye for now. I walk back into the studio, in awe of the emptiness here.

Epilogue

*Whoever delves into mysticism cannot help
but stumble, as it is written: "This stumbling
block is in your hand." You cannot grasp these
things unless you stumble over them.*

KABBALAH

Dusk arrives once again. The studio is empty. I light a candle and sit at the stone bowl, tracing the rim of this empty circle with my hand, slowly, very slowly, so that I can feel the tool marks with my fingertips. Now I see others sitting with me around the bowl. Each one is vivid, present.

> May the emptiness within this vessel
>   be a source from which
>   we can see more clearly.

Now my fingers stumble into a place where a tiny chip has fallen away, marking an indentation. Putting my finger in this hollow, I trace a dark and delicate line, a fissure, that moves away from the wounded place. I must enter this crevice, this sacred imperfection. My heart follows the fault line into the density of the stone, into the density of this vessel, within this studio, this home, this nation, becoming our world. How will this crack in the container, this woundedness that is inherent in wholeness, call toward and receive the light of unbounded, conscious forces, strengthening our vessel? How will this same crack release the uncontained darkness of unconscious forces, threatening to shatter the whole of our fragile humanity?

> May the quality of consciousness
> that is emerging collectively
> within our world
> outweigh the quantity of unconsciousness
> that suffers on our planet.
> May all suffering become compassion.
> May we be ready, may we be able.

The discipline of Authentic Movement is one more evolving embodied awareness practice, one more opportunity for participating in creating a world which must endure.

JANET ADLER
JULY 2002

Epigraph Source Notes

Preface

Rumi, *Like This,* trans. Coleman Barks (Coleman Barks, 1990), 30.

John Martin, *The Modern Dance* (New York: Dance Horizons, 1933), 59.

The Individual Body

Satprem, *Sri Aurobindo or the Adventure of Consciousness* (New York: India Library Society, 1984), 185.

Daniel Matt, trans. *The Essential Kabbalah: The Heart of Jewish Mysticism* (San Francisco: HarperSanFrancisco, 1996), 67.

Lukardis of Oberweimar, Life by an anonymous author, published in Analecta Bollandiana, vol. xviii (1899) 314.

Arthur Green, *Seek My Face, Speak My Name* (Northvale, New Jersey: Jason Aronson, 1992), 65.

Daniel Ladinsky, trans. *The Gift: Poems by Hafiz* (New York: Penguin Arkana, 1999), p. 99.

D. T. Suzuki, *The Awakening of Zen* (Boulder: Prajna Press, 1980), 52-53.

Satprem, *Sri Aurobindo or the Adventure of Consciousness* (New York: India Library Society, 1984), 71.

The Collective Body

Marion L. Matics, trans. *Entering the Path of Enlightenment: The Bodhicaryavatara of the Buddhist Poet Santiveda* (New York: n.p., 1970), 202-204.

Stephen Mitchell, ed. *The Enlightened Heart: An Anthology of Sacred Poetry* (New York: Harper Perennial, 1989), 104.

Daniel Matt, trans. *The Essential Kabbalah: The Heart of Jewish Mysticism* (San Francisco: HarperSanFrancisco, 1996), 93.

The Conscious Body

D. C. Lau, *Confucius: The Analects,* trans. Lun Yu (London: Penguin, 1979), 76.

Lao-tzu, *Tao te Ching,* trans. Stephen Mitchell (New York: HarperCollins, 1988), 45.

Antonio de Nicholas, *St. John of the Cross: Alchemist of the Soul* (New York: Paragon House, 1989), 52.

Rudolf Laban, *A Life for Dance* (London: MacDonald & Evans, 1975), 89.

Ajit Mookerjee, *Kundalini: The Arousal of the Inner Energy* (New York: Destiny Books, 1982), 77.

Daniel Matt, trans. *The Essential Kabbalah: The Heart of Jewish Mysticism* (San Francisco: HarperSanFrancisco, 1996), 163.

Books of Related Interest

ARCHING BACKWARD
The Mystical Initiation of a Contemporary Woman
by Janet Adler

THE BODY OF LIFE
Creating New Pathways for Sensory Awareness and Fluid Movement
by Thomas Hanna

THE BODY HAS ITS REASONS
Self-Awareness Through Conscious Movement
by Therese Bertherat and Carol Bernstein

THE ALEXANDER TECHNIQUE
How to Use Your Body without Stress
by Wilfred Barlow, M.D.

SACRED WOMAN, SACRED DANCE
Awakening Spirituality Through Movement and Ritual
by Iris J. Stewart

EARTHWALKS FOR BODY AND SPIRIT
Exercises to Restore Our Sacred Bond with the Earth
by James Endredy

SHAPESHIFTING
Shamanic Techniques for Global and Personal Transformation
by John Perkins

TRANSFORMING YOUR DRAGONS
How to Turn Fear Patterns into Personal Power
by José Stevens

Inner Traditions • Bear & Company
P.O. Box 388 • Rochester, VT 05767
1-800-246-8648
www.InnerTraditions.com

Or contact your local bookseller